Women's Group Treatment for Substance Use Disorder is an evidence-based, easy-to-learn program that is specifically tailored to address issues of critical importance to women suffering with alcohol and drug use disorders. It is flexible and can be delivered as a stand-alone treatment or in the context of a larger treatment program. The therapist can create personalized treatment plans using the modules most relevant to the individual patient. The Therapist Guide and Client Workbook are tremendously useful. I highly recommend this program—it should be a part of the armamentarium for anyone treating women with substance use disorders.

—Kathleen T. Brady, M.D., Ph.D., Distinguished University Professor, Medical University of South Carolina, Director, South Carolina Clinical and Translational Research Institute

Drs. Epstein and McCrady's Therapist Guide and Client Workbook to help women with substance use disorders fills a longstanding and critical need in the treatment field. The materials are comprehensive and easy to use, explaining the why and how of treatment. Therapists are guided step by step through each treatment session, and clients are offered instructive handouts and worksheets to practice new coping skills week by week. This tested, flexible, and collaborative approach is an invaluable resource for both therapists and clients to begin and sustain women's recovery.

—Christine Timko, Ph.D., Senior Research Career Scientist, Health Services Research and Development, Department of Veterans Affairs; Clinical Professor (Affiliated), Department of Psychiatry and Behavioral Sciences, Stanford University School of Medicine

It's rare to feel empowered by reading a therapist's manual, but this one had that effect. The authors' integration of skills backed by solid research evidence with attentiveness to issues commonly faced by women results in a supportive, easily implemented program that is applicable in a variety of clinical and recovery support settings. The focus on self-confidence and self-care in every session, and the balance of emphasis on empathic validation and motivation for change, make this a powerful approach to working with women with substance use and co-occurring mental health disorders.

—Annie Peters, Ph.D., Director of Research and Education, National Association of Addiction Treatment Providers

Women's Group Treatment for Substance Use Disorder

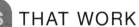 **✔ TREATMENTS THAT WORK**

Women's Group Treatment for Substance Use Disorder

Evidence-Based Cognitive Behavioral Therapy

THERAPIST GUIDE

ELIZABETH E. EPSTEIN

BARBARA S. MCCRADY

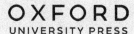
OXFORD
UNIVERSITY PRESS

OXFORD
UNIVERSITY PRESS

Oxford University Press is a department of the University of Oxford. It furthers
the University's objective of excellence in research, scholarship, and education
by publishing worldwide. Oxford is a registered trade mark of Oxford University
Press in the UK and certain other countries.

Published in the United States of America by Oxford University Press
198 Madison Avenue, New York, NY 10016, United States of America.

Library of Congress Cataloging-in-Publication Data
Names: Epstein, Elizabeth E., editor. | McCrady, Barbara S., editor.
Title: Women's group treatment for substance use disorder :
evidence-based cognitive behavioral therapy. Therapist guide /
[edited by] Elizabeth E. Epstein, Barbara S. McCrady.
Description: New York, NY : Oxford University Press, [2023] |
Series: Treatments that work | Includes bibliographical references and index. |
Identifiers: LCCN 2022054554 (print) | LCCN 2022054555 (ebook) |
ISBN 9780197655085 (paperback) | ISBN 9780197655108 (epub) |
ISBN 9780197655115 (ebook)
Subjects: LCSH: Women—Substance use. | Women—Alcohol use. |
Alcoholism—Treatment. | Substance abuse—Treatment. |
Cognitive therapy—Problems, exercises, etc. |
Group psychotherapy—Problems, exercises, etc.
Classification: LCC RC564.5.W65 W673 2023 (print) |
LCC RC564.5.W65 (ebook) | DDC 362.29082—dc23/eng/20221223
LC record available at https://lccn.loc.gov/2022054554
LC ebook record available at https://lccn.loc.gov/2022054555

DOI: 10.1093/med-psych/9780197655085.001.0001

Printed by Marquis Book Printing, Canada

To my family, to Barbara, and to David.

—EEE

To my sister Judi, an extraordinary woman.

—BSM

Stunning developments in healthcare have taken place over the last several years, but many of our widely accepted interventions and strategies in mental health and behavioral medicine have been brought into question by research evidence as not only lacking benefit but, perhaps, even inducing harm (Barlow, 2010). Other strategies have been proven effective using the best current standards of evidence, resulting in broad-based recommendations to make these practices more available to the public (McHugh & Barlow, 2010). Several recent developments are behind this revolution. First, we have arrived at a much deeper understanding of pathology, both psychological and physical, which has led to the development of new, more precisely targeted interventions. Second, our research methodologies have improved substantially, such that we have reduced threats to internal and external validity, making the outcomes more directly applicable to clinical situations. Third, governments around the world and health care systems and policymakers have decided that the quality of care should improve, that it should be evidence-based, and that it is in the public's interest to ensure that this happens (Barlow, 2004; Institute of Medicine, 2001, 2015; McHugh & Barlow, 2010).

Of course, the major stumbling block for clinicians everywhere is the accessibility of newly developed evidence-based psychological interventions. Workshops and books can go only so far in acquainting responsible and conscientious practitioners with the latest behavioral health care practices and their applicability to individual patients. This series, Treatments *That Work*, is devoted to communicating these exciting new interventions to clinicians on the frontlines of practice.

The manuals and workbooks in this series contain step-by-step detailed procedures for assessing and treating specific problems and diagnoses. But this series also goes beyond the books and manuals by providing ancillary materials that will approximate the supervisory process in assisting practitioners in the implementation of these procedures in their practice.

In our emerging health care system, the growing consensus is that evidence-based practice offers the most responsible course of action for the mental health professional. All behavioral health care clinicians deeply desire to provide the best possible care for their patients. In this series, our aim is to close the dissemination and information gap and make that possible.

Based on scientific evidence accumulated over 25 years of National Institutes of Health (NIH)-funded studies, this Therapist Guide focuses on women with alcohol use disorder (AUD) and other substance use disorders (SUDs), to address the unique problems and treatment needs they face. Women with AUD/SUD have different etiology, mortality, relapse antecedents, clinical presentation, and course of the disorders than men, requiring specialized techniques and interventions. This is a cognitive behavioral, motivation-enhancing protocol for therapists to deliver in inpatient or intensive outpatient settings or as a stand-alone weekly outpatient treatment. The protocol is presented in group therapy modality, but can be easily adapted for individual therapy. Interventions over 12 weekly sessions help women become abstinent and prevent relapse to drinking or drug use, and achieve improvement in secondary outcomes: quality of life, depression and anxiety, self-care, wellness, and self-compassion, shame, trauma symptoms, coping skills, healthy relationships, self-confidence, autonomy, and emotional reactivity.

The Therapist Guide includes step-by-step cognitive behavioral therapy (CBT) interventions to address: ambivalence around changing drinking and drug use; abstinence planning; self-monitoring of triggers, cravings, and alcohol/drug use; behavior chains; handling triggers and high-risk situations; drink/drug refusal; dealing with cravings; alcohol-related thoughts; reinforcing abstinence; and relapse prevention. General coping skills such as problem-solving, assertiveness training, wellness behaviors, and communication training are taught and practiced. Additional female-specific interventions address social network support for abstinence; building healthy, supportive relationships; and mood problems. In the group therapy modality, the therapy protocol harnesses peer support, shared wisdom, and universality of experience to accelerate positive change in desired outcomes.

David H. Barlow, Editor-in-Chief
Treatments *That Work*
Boston, MA

References

Barlow, D. H. (2004). Psychological treatments. *American Psychologist, 59*, 869–878.

Barlow, D. H. (2010). Negative effects from psychological treatments: A perspective. *American Psychologist, 65*(2), 13–20.

Institute of Medicine. (2001). *Crossing the quality chasm: A new health system for the 21st century*. National Academy Press.

Institute of Medicine. (2015). *Psychosocial interventions for mental and substance use disorders: A framework for establishing evidence-based standards*. National Academies Press.

McHugh, R. K., & Barlow, D. H. (2010). Dissemination and implementation of evidence-based psychological interventions: A review of current efforts. *American Psychologist, 65*(2), 73–84.

Contents

Acknowledgments

The authors are grateful to the National Institute on Alcohol Abuse and Alcoholism for funding that supported their research, and to NIAAA Project Officers Dr. Angela Martinelli and Dr. Brett Hagman. This work could not have been done without our phenomenal research team who helped us develop and refine this treatment program, and the many study participants and clients who trusted us to help them navigate a path through alcohol and drug problems. We also are deeply appreciative of David Fenichel for reading, editing, proofreading, and generally improving each session. We would like to thank Kate Scheinman for her editorial work. We are grateful to Sarah Harrington, Oxford University Press Executive Editor, who was unfailingly supportive and helpful in providing expert and wise guidance at every turn.

CHAPTER 1

Introductory Information for Therapists

Why Women-Specific Treatment for Alcohol and Other Substance Use Disorders?

Women with alcohol use disorder (AUD) and other substance use disorders (SUDs) have different etiology, mortality, relapse antecedents, clinical presentation, and course of the disorders than men with AUD/SUD (see Epstein & Menges, 2013; Epstein et al., 2018b). For instance, relative to men, women report higher comorbidity of mood, anxiety, post-traumatic stress, eating, and personality disorders (Rosenthal, 2013), and women are likely to drink alone, in secrecy, daily, in response to relationship difficulties (Zweig et al., 2009), and in response to negative emotional triggers (Abulseoud et al., 2013). Women tend to have social networks that include family members and romantic partners with SUD (Leonard & Homish, 2008) who do not support recovery (McCrady, 2004). Many relapse antecedents are more prevalent in women than men, including being alone, negative affect, interpersonal problems, and relationship distress (Walitzer & Dearing, 2006). Mediators of treatment on AUD outcomes also may differ by gender; mechanisms of change generally relevant to women likely include alleviation of negative affect, enhanced coping skills and self-care, improved interpersonal functioning (Velasquez & Stotts, 2003), and greater emotion regulation (Ashley et al., 2003; Timko et al., 2005). Gender differences in clinical presentation of addiction, relapse antecedents, and mediators suggest that treatments tailored to women's concerns may enhance access to treatment and yield more positive outcomes than gender-neutral programs. Treatment utilization for alcohol use problems is lower for women than for men. Women may be more likely to seek help if single-gender treatment is offered (Cucciare et al., 2013; Lewis et al., 2016); however, female-segregated treatments have been found to be efficacious only if they include female-specific programming (Epstein & Menges, 2013; Holzhauer et al., 2020a).

These documented gender differences, increasing rates of AUD and other SUDs in women (Grant et al., 2015), and the accelerated negative impact of AUD/SUD on women's health all underscore the need to provide female-tailored treatment options that enhance accessibility, engagement, and efficacy of existing treatments that originally were developed with predominantly male samples. Women with AUD face particular barriers to seeking help, and fewer women (15%) than men (23%) with AUD seek treatment for it in their lifetime (Alvanzo et al., 2014). Widespread availability of female-only treatment settings that include evidence-based female-specific interventions and content is likely to increase treatment utilization and enhance outcomes for women with SUD, but this currently is lacking (Heslin et al., 2015).

Women's Group Treatment for Substance Use Disorder: Evidence-Based Cognitive Behavioral Therapy—Therapist Guide (along with the accompanying Client Workbook) provides an evidence-based, cognitive behavioral, easy-to-learn, easy-to-use program for therapists to employ. The program is flexible in delivery—it can be used as a stand-alone weekly outpatient group, or offered in the context of a comprehensive inpatient or intensive outpatient AUD/SUD treatment program. The Therapist Guide and Client Workbook can also be easily adapted for individual therapy. Sessions and interventions/topics within sessions are clearly delineated and can be delivered in the order presented in the guide, or can be extracted as needed to create a personalized treatment plan for each type and/or membership of group, or for each client in individual therapy. This female-specific program is evidence-based, having been developed over the course of three 5-year National Institute on Alcohol Abuse and Alcoholism (NIAAA)-funded randomized trials (Epstein et al., 2018a, 2018b; McCrady et al., 2016). This program provides an evidence-based female-only/female-specific content option for outpatient practitioners, SUD inpatient and outpatient programs, and primary care clinics to enhance treatment access, engagement, and outcomes for SUD and secondary outcomes such as mood problems, independence, and coping skills for women with AUD and other drug use problems.

This Therapist Guide includes introductory material, an assessment chapter, and 12 therapy sessions written for women-only group delivery, but these can be easily adapted for use with a female client in individual therapy. The treatment can be a stand-alone weekly outpatient treatment protocol for women with risky substance use or SUD, or can be embedded into existing inpatient or intensive outpatient programs for SUD. Therapists employ a non-confrontational, collaborative style consistent with the spirit of motivational interviewing (MI) (Miller & Rollnick, 2013) used in high-quality cognitive behavioral treatment (CBT). All language, examples, vignettes, worksheets, and illustrations are female-specific. The treatment program includes core CBT elements to treat SUD; general coping skills; female-specific interventions; and important women's issues and themes of autonomy and self-care that are integrated into each session via discussion and illustrative material.

Regarding terminology, throughout this Therapist Guide and the companion Client Workbook, the term "alcohol use disorder (AUD)" is used in instances related specifically to problem alcohol use; the term "other drug use problems" is used to refer to non-alcohol drugs; and "substance use disorder (SUD)" is an umbrella term to cover both alcohol and other drugs. The word "client" is used rather than "patient," but these two words have the same meaning—the recipient of this treatment.

Goals and Purpose of Therapy

The treatment is designed to help women become abstinent and prevent relapse to drinking or drug use, as well as to improve secondary outcomes: an improved quality of life, a decrease in depression and anxiety, increased self-care and self-compassion, decreased shame, decreased trauma symptoms, enhanced coping skills, healthier relationships, enhanced self-confidence, and decreased emotional reactivity to others. These primary and secondary outcomes define what can be considered a female-specific variant of contemporary definitions of "recovery" (Betty Ford, 2007; El-Guebaly, 2012; Witkiewitz & Tucker, 2020).

Epidemiology

Use of alcohol and other drugs is common in the United States; among women, 62% have consumed alcohol in the past year, compared to 72% of men (White, 2020). Drug use is less common, with 16.2% of women and 22.7% of men reporting illicit use of any drug in the past year. Marijuana is by far the most commonly used drug, with 12.4% of women and 18.4% of men reporting use in the past year (National Institute on Drug Abuse [NIDA], 2020).

Unfortunately, use of alcohol or any other drug has the potential to lead to adverse consequences and development of an SUD ranging in severity from mild (two or three symptoms) to moderate (four or five symptoms) to severe (six or more of 11 symptoms). Eleven criteria for SUD from the fifth edition of the *Diagnostic and Statistical Manual of Mental Disorders* (*DSM-5*; American Psychiatric Association, 2013) are paraphrased here: loss of control of the amount of substance used or time spent using; worry about drinking/using drug too much and/or failed attempts to cut down or quit; 10 or more hours per week spent acquiring, using, or getting over the effects of a substance; strong craving; inability to meet obligations because of the substance use; continuing to use alcohol or drugs even though they are problematic for social or interpersonal functioning; using the substance in lieu of other prior social, job-related, or recreational activities; using a substance in situations where use may increase risk of physical injury; knowing that the substance is causing or worsening a medical or emotional problem and continuing to use it anyway; developing physiological tolerance; and experiencing a withdrawal syndrome after reducing or stopping the substance use or using the substance to prevent withdrawal. An AUD or SUD may be classified as in partial remission or full remission; remission may be early (at least 3 months) or sustained (1 year or more) (American Psychiatric Association, 2013).

Rates of past-year AUD are 10.4% among women and 17.6% among men; for lifetime AUD, rates are 22.7% among women and 36% among men (Grant et al., 2015). Past-year prevalence for any non-alcohol SUD among women is 3% and for men 4.9%, while lifetime prevalence of non-alcohol SUD is 7.7% for women and 12.3% for men. There has been a steep trajectory of gender convergence over the last 20 years in both alcohol and other drug use and disorders (Grant et al., 2015, 2016; McHugh et al., 2018). For instance, from 2000 to 2013, rates of past 12-month AUD (*DSM-IV-TR*; American Psychiatric Association, 2000) abuse or dependence among women increased by 83.7% (from 4.9% to 9%) while the rate of AUD for men increased by 34.7% (from 12.4% to 16.7%; Grant et al., 2015). In general, non-Hispanic whites have higher rates of AUD and SUD than Hispanics, and, among racial groups, American Indians/Alaska Natives have the highest rate of AUD and SUD (Grant et al., 2016). In addition, persons who identify as sexual minorities are more likely to engage in binge drinking, with twice the rates among lesbian or bisexual women as women who identify as heterosexual (National Survey of Drug Using Households, 2019).

Contemporary Neuroscience Conceptualization of AUD and SUD

The NIAAA defines AUD as a "chronic relapsing brain disease characterized by an impaired ability to stop or control alcohol use despite adverse social, occupational, or health consequences" (NIAAA, 2017, pp. 16–17; NIAAA, 2021b, p. 1). The NIDA defines SUD as a "chronic, relapsing disorder characterized by compulsive drug seeking and use despite adverse consequences" (NIDA, 2019). The brain disease presents in a cycle of three stages (Volkow & Koob, 2019):

- "Binge/intoxication" is a loss of control of drinking/drug use involving structures in the basal ganglia, considered the "reward center" of the brain. Alcohol/drug triggers repeatedly activate the reward center, leading to increased salience of alcohol/drug cues and habit formation by repeated associations of cues with reinforcing effects of substances, via changes in the striatum.
- "Withdrawal/negative affect" occurs when repeated periods between drinking/drug episodes create both a reward deficit and enhanced stress reaction in the amygdala.
- "Preoccupation/anticipation" arises from irregularities in the prefrontal cortex, resulting in deficits in cognitive control over alcohol/drug-seeking behavior (Koob, 2013).

There is some preliminary evidence for sex differences in the neurobiology and vulnerability to the onset of problem drinking, development of AUD/SUD, and relapse (see Flores-Bonilla & Richardson, 2020; McHugh et al., 2018).

Course

Women have a "risk-severity paradox" (White, 2020): They metabolize alcohol less efficiently than men and may use lesser amounts of alcohol or drugs than men but experience greater harm/negative consequences. Women who drink heavily are at heightened risk for adverse medical consequences, including hangovers, liver inflammation, progression of alcoholic liver disease, cardiovascular disease, and some kinds of cancers (see McCrady et al., 2020). Risk of all these adverse consequences is accelerated with age. Women who use other drugs may be more vulnerable to cardiovascular effects, exposure to sexually transmitted diseases, and death from drug overdoses (NIDA, 2020). Use of alcohol or other drugs during pregnancy places a woman at higher risk of miscarriage and places the developing fetus at risk of premature birth, low birth weight, and fetal alcohol spectrum disorder after exposure to alcohol, or neonatal abstinence syndrome after exposure to opioids or some other drugs (e.g., benzodiazepines, barbiturates). The period from the age of onset of regular drinking or drug use to the development of AUD or SUD is shorter for women than men (often called a "telescoping effect").

Women with AUD or SUD often have co-occurring mental health disorders and are at heightened risk for being victims of intimate partner violence. National survey data suggest that the rates of mood and anxiety disorders are 1.5 to 2 times greater in women with AUD compared to men with AUD and that comorbidities may be higher in a treatment-seeking population. Women in treatment also report very high lifetime rates of trauma and abuse, which may be physical, sexual, or emotional, with concomitant high rates of post-traumatic stress disorder (PTSD) (reviewed in McCrady et al., 2020). Many women entering treatment are currently in relationships that are emotionally or physically abusive (reviewed in McCrady et al., 2020).

Most AUD and SUD treatments were originally developed for men. Now that the literature has made it clear that women with AUD/SUD have specific and unique clinical characteristics, treatment programs should be designed to reduce perceived barriers and facilitate positive outcomes for women. In addition to the unique presenting problems and concerns of women described above, there are several additional reasons for women-only groups with content tailored to the concerns of women: (a) barriers that women experience in seeking AUD or SUD treatment; (b) the clinical context of women-only versus mixed gender groups; and (c) the unique content of women-specific treatment.

Barriers to Treatment Entry Unique to Women

Women experience unique barriers to seeking or receiving AUD or SUD treatment (see McCrady et al., 2020). Stigma about AUD and SUD is amplified for women, which contributes to anxiety, depression, shame, and hiding their alcohol or drug use from family and friends. Women-only treatment may mitigate shame-based obstacles to treatment entry. Families often are less supportive of women than men seeking treatment. Women with AUD or SUD often have an intimate partner who also is a heavy user of alcohol or drugs and may not support her efforts to change, or may even actively oppose a reduction in her drinking/drug use. A supportive group therapy environment with other women is designed to amplify existing social support networks for clients.

Women often have primary responsibility for the care of their children and can find it difficult to balance these responsibilities with their own treatment needs, and also may be concerned about the potential involvement of child protective services should they seek treatment. Therapists must walk a fine line between developing the trust of women with children and adhering to ethical and legal responsibilities to report potential child abuse. Generally, a useful approach is to align with the client's wish to keep her children safe.

Treatment Context for Women: Why Gender-Segregated Treatment?

Mixed-gender groups and settings may be particularly uncomfortable for women with a history of sexual or physical trauma (Lewis et al., 2016). Also, literature about the interactional dominance of men in mixed-gender settings such as therapy groups suggests that women may be hesitant to participate fully in therapy groups that include both men and women (Greenfield & Pirard, 2009). Confrontational treatment approaches may be incongruent with a woman's clinical needs. Women-only groups are likely to enhance treatment access and engagement, and provision of female-specific content in the groups enhances outcomes.

Treatment Content for Women

Since the National Institutes of Health mandate in 1994 that biomedical research include female participants in clinical research, a substantive body of literature has emerged describing unique aspects of AUD and SUD among women (see Epstein & Menges, 2013). This information has guided development of female-specific topic areas to address in treatment, such as family support or resistance to change; partner or family substance use; intimate partner violence; shame and stigma about alcohol or drug use; coping with negative emotions; and co-occurring disorders. Throughout treatment, therapists should encourage a sense of agency and self-determination, communicate respect and appreciation for their clients' strengths, and support women's valuing of relationships and interconnectedness while at the same time helping them recognize self-destructive interpersonal patterns (Ashley et al., 2003; Substance Abuse and Mental Health Services Administration, 2013).

For women with AUD or SUD, additional service needs might include support for detoxification; treatment for associated medical conditions; evaluation for psychotropic medication; prenatal care; or linkage to social welfare programs such as Medicaid, Medicare, food stamps, or housing or food assistance. Neither a single therapist nor a treatment program can provide all of these services, but having a well-vetted list of referral resources may also make it easier for a woman to access and continue in treatment and to achieve positive outcomes.

The Women's CBT Group for SUD—the treatment program presented in this Therapist Guide and the companion Client Workbook—was found in NIAAA-funded randomized clinical trials (RCTs) to be equivalent to evidence-based control treatments in alcohol use outcomes and should enhance accessibility of AUD and SUD treatments for women. It also yields positive secondary outcomes for depression and anxiety (Epstein et al., 2018a, 2018b), cardiovascular function (Buckman et al., 2019), health behaviors (Bold et al., 2017), drug use (Epstein et al., 2015), and overall quality of life (Bold et al., 2017). One study compared a stand-alone, weekly 12-session outpatient individual-modality Female-Specific Cognitive Behavioral Therapy (FS-CBT) to similar evidence-based gender-neutral CBT for AUD (Epstein et al., 2018a). Women in both treatment conditions (N = 99) were highly engaged in the treatment; were very satisfied with the treatment; significantly reduced their drinking during the 4 months of treatment; and maintained their positive drinking outcomes over the next year. They also improved and maintained gains in other areas of life functioning, such as depression, anxiety, autonomy, and sociotropy. The FS-CBT treatment was equally effective to the evidence-based gender-neutral one. A subsequent NIAAA-funded RCT compared the individual-modality FS-CBT treatment to a group therapy format with the same content (i.e., the Women's Group Therapy for SUD) in a "pure comparison" design (N = 138 women with AUD)—identical 12-session, outpatient, weekly manual-guided treatment except the treatment was delivered in women-only groups versus individual therapy (Epstein et al., 2018b). Both FS-CBT treatment modalities (individual and group therapy) resulted in significant positive changes in drinking, depression, anxiety, coping skills, self-confidence, interpersonal functioning, and self-care during the 4 months of outpatient treatment that were maintained for at least 1 year following treatment. Client satisfaction for both the individual and group modalities was very high. Importantly, cost-effectiveness analyses favored the group format (Olmstead et al., 2019).

For the group- versus individual-modality FS-CBT randomized trial, of 341 alcohol-dependent women screened, seven women (2%) were excluded due to past-month physiological dependence on other drugs. The remaining sample of women had extensive lifetime drug use histories: 87% had used at least one illicit drug in their lifetime, and 15% had used at least one illicit drug in the month prior to alcohol treatment. Lifetime and past-year use of illicit drugs was associated with younger age, but up to 89% of women had used illicit drugs in their lifetime. Cannabis was the most typically used other drug and was most strongly related to their pattern of alcohol use and outcome. Lifetime rates of tobacco use (80%) also exceeded lifetime rates in community samples of women. Almost one-third of the women (29%) had been daily tobacco smokers in the year before treatment (Bold et al., 2020). Treatment for alcohol use was associated with reductions in drug use during treatment as well. However, women who continued to use illicit drugs during treatment had worse alcohol outcomes. Since the alcohol interventions in the tested female-specific CBT group for AUD are equally applicable to illicit drug use and nicotine use behavioral, the Women's CBT Group described in this manual includes non-alcohol drug information. Interventions are also compatible with behavioral nicotine cessation programs. Contemporary best practice treatment for SUD, AUD, and nicotine cessation includes adjunct medication-assisted treatment (MAT), which is discussed in Chapter 3.

Our research team piloted a rolling-admission format of group FS-CBT using a within-subject pre-post study design. Women entered the group at any session and attended as many sessions as they wanted; they attended a mean of 15 sessions (SD = 13). Fifty-three percent of the women were continuously abstinent. Growth curve analyses showed significantly decreased drinking intensity and cravings and improved mood. Our team also piloted a 12-session rolling-admission group for female Veterans using Women's CBT Group for SUD at a SUD outpatient specialty care unit at a Veterans Administration (VA) site. Over 8 months, 69% of women referred attended at least one group session. In an exit interview, participants rated several treatment elements as helpful or greatly helpful, including: the group format, support of other group members, learning about alcohol effects on women, managing strong negative emotion, the focus on taking care of yourself, empowerment, women's issues, and having only women in the group.

Research on moderators of outcome (Longabaugh et al., 2013) has elucidated the importance of heterogeneity within samples and helped to refine female-specific treatments. For example, findings that anxiety pre-treatment and depression pre- and post-treatment predicted poorer drinking outcomes for women (Haver & Gjestad, 2005) suggest the importance of including interventions to alleviate depression and anxiety in female-specific AUD treatment. Using data from our female-specific versus gender-neutral RCT, Holzhauer et al. (2017) found that women who enter treatment struggling with negative affect may respond particularly well to the targeted interventions for depression, anxiety, and emotion regulation. Hayaki et al. (2020) found that phase of the menstrual cycle also has an impact on drinking. Hallgren et al. (2019) used daily data from the individual versus group female-specific RCT and found that women who initiated abstinence during treatment showed marked improvements in two key hypothesized mechanisms of change—abstinence self-efficacy and coping skills—during the week that they initiated abstinence. Hallgren et al. (2016) also found that daily alcohol cravings decreased in relation to the initiation of abstinence in men and women in outpatient CBT for AUD. Using a statistical approach to simultaneously examine change among several hypothesized mechanisms of change, Holzhauer et al. (2020b) compared pathways to drinking reduction among women in gender-neutral versus FS-CBT. Across treatments, women changed their drinking via increased coping skills, self-efficacy for abstinence, and increased autonomy. For women in FS-CBT, changes in drinking also occurred through decreases in sociotropy and increases in social support for abstinence.

Conclusion

Women with AUD and other SUDs have unique problems and treatment needs that are best served with treatments tailored to those needs. Over the past 30 years, we have been developing, refining, and rigorously testing treatments to address these needs. This Therapist Guide represents the culmination of these efforts and provides a detailed guide for therapists who want to use the latest scientific evidence to provide clinically sensitive and effective treatment to their female clients with AUD and other SUDs.

CHAPTER 2

What Is Women's CBT Group for SUD?

Overview of the Treatment

This treatment covers core cognitive behavioral therapy (CBT) motivational and skills-based elements to treat alcohol use disorder (AUD) and substance use disorder (SUD), including a detailed assessment of alcohol and drug use and related problems, motivational enhancement to reduce ambivalence around changing drinking and drug use, goal-setting, abstinence planning, self-monitoring, functional analysis (behavior chains), self-management planning, drink/drug refusal, dealing with cravings, coping with alcohol-related thoughts, and relapse prevention, as well as general coping skills such as problem-solving and communication training.

The Therapist Guide also includes a set of female-specific coping skills, each linked to an issue of particular importance for women with AUD or SUD:

1. Psychoeducation about women and alcohol or drug use
2. Enhancing social support for abstinence by increasing sober members in the social network and coping effectively with drug users or heavy drinkers in the existing social network
3. Interpersonal functioning, including choosing and connecting with others in respectful, nurturing relationships; increasing autonomy, self-confidence, and assertiveness; and decreasing negative emotional reactivity to others
4. Well-being and self-care: nurturing oneself emotionally through self-compassion and behaviorally through healthy habits (for example, exercise, leisure, and nutrition)
5. Identifying and coping with mood problems such as depression and anxiety, negative affect, anger, shame, trauma reactions, and emotion dysregulation.

In addition, two thematic women's issues are integrated into each session via discussion and illustrative material:

1. Enhanced sense of autonomy (self-confidence to cope independently, emphasizing the woman as an active agent in her own life to increase empowerment) and decreased sociotropy (being less emotionally and behaviorally reactive to others' negative behavior and perceived expectations)

2. Self-care for personal well-being through activities such as exercise, a supportive social network, leisure activities, and healthy nutrition; setting boundaries with others; and developing new thinking patterns that yield more self-compassionate and fewer shame thoughts.

The session-by-session outline for this manual is shown in Table 2.1, with interventions broken down into categories of routine interventions done at every session, alcohol- and drug-specific coping skills interventions, and female-specific interventions.

CBT for Alcohol/Drug Use and Related Problems

The treatment we present in this Therapist Guide is evidence-based CBT modified to integrate women-specific themes and content. CBT derives partially from behavioral theories such as classical and operant conditioning and social modeling, and partially from cognitive therapy (Beck & Haigh, 2014), and addresses reciprocal interactions among triggers (situations/events), thoughts, feelings, and behavior (see Carroll, 1999; Mastroleo & Monti, 2013). CBT interventions are organized around three major elements in this program:

1. Motivational enhancement to change alcohol and drug use behavior

2. Alcohol/drug-focused behavioral and cognitive coping skills to attain abstinence and prevent relapse

3. Skills to address common female-specific challenges among women with SUD, such as management of anger, interpersonal function, trauma reactions, anxiety, depression, emotion regulation, shame, and assertiveness.

Table 2.1. Women's CBT Group for SUD

Routine Interventions: Alcohol/Drug	Alcohol/Drug-Related Interventions	Female-Specific Interventions
Session 1: Orientation, Daily Monitoring, and Abstinence Plans		
▩ Blood alcohol level (BAL)/drug screen ▩ Therapist introduction and agenda setting ▩ Introduction of group members ▩ Workbook, treatment requirements, group contract ▩ Round robin check-in: review of self-monitoring and homework, review of abstinence plans for continuing group members ▩ Farewell to members leaving the group ▩ Homework	▩ Feedback from intake assessment ▩ Introduction to self-monitoring ▩ Abstinence plan (optional) and/or possible problem areas (optional) ▩ Anticipating high-risk situations	▩ Treatment rationale and psychoeducation on female alcohol and drug problems; importance of homework and attendance
Session 2: Triggers and Behavior Chains		
▩ BAL/drug screen ▩ Introductions and agenda setting ▩ Round robin check-in: review of self-monitoring and homework, review of abstinence plans (if needed) ▩ Homework	▩ Behavior chains/identifying triggers ▩ Anticipating high-risk situations	
Session 3: Presence of Heavy Drinkers/Drug Users in Social Network; Self-Management Plans		
▩ BAL/drug screen ▩ Introductions and agenda setting ▩ Round robin check-in: review of self- monitoring and homework ▩ Update abstinence plan ▩ Homework	▩ Self-management planning ▩ Anticipating high-risk situations	▩ Presence of heavy drinkers/drug users in social network ▩ Assessing the impact of social network on change efforts

(continued)

15

Table 2.1. Continued

Routine Interventions: Alcohol/Drug	Alcohol/Drug-Related Interventions	Female-Specific Interventions

Session 4: Enhancing Motivation to Change and Increasing Positive Consequences of Abstinence

- BAL/drug screen
- Introductions and agenda setting
- Round robin check-in: review of self-monitoring and homework
- Update abstinence plan
- Homework

- Decisional matrix and rearranging positive consequences of abstinence
- Anticipating high-risk situations

Session 5: Well-Being and Self-Care

- BAL/drug screen
- Introductions and agenda setting
- Round robin check-in: review of self-monitoring and homework
- Update abstinence plan
- Homework

- Anticipating high-risk situations

- Well-being
- Self-care (self-compassion and behavioral self-care)

Session 6: Identifying Anxiety, Depression, Trauma; Coping with Cravings

- BAL/drug screen
- Introductions and agenda setting
- Round robin check-in: review of self-monitoring and homework
- Homework

- Coping with cravings to drink/use drugs
- Anticipating high-risk situations

- What is anxiety?
- What is depression?
- What is trauma?

Session 7: Affect and Mood Management

- BAL/drug screen
- Introductions and agenda setting
- Round robin check-in: review of self-monitoring and homework
- Homework

- Anticipating high-risk situations

- Cognitive and behavioral strategies to manage negative emotions, moods, and stress reactivity

Table 2.1. Continued

Routine Interventions: Alcohol/Drug	Alcohol/Drug-Related Interventions	Female-Specific Interventions
Session 8: Connecting with Others, Dealing with Alcohol/Drug-Related Thoughts		
▪ BAL/drug screen	▪ Dealing with alcohol/drug-related thoughts	▪ Connecting with others: improving social support for abstinence
▪ Introductions and agenda setting	▪ Anticipating high-risk situations	
▪ Round robin check-in: review of self- monitoring and homework		
▪ Homework		
Session 9: Assertiveness Training and Drink/Drug Refusal		
▪ BAL/drug screen	▪ Drink/drug refusal training	▪ Assertiveness training and effective communication
▪ Introductions and agenda setting	▪ Anticipating high-risk situations	
▪ Round robin check-in: review of self-monitoring and homework		
▪ Homework		
Session 10: Anger Management; Relapse Prevention I: Seemingly Irrelevant Decisions		
▪ BAL/drug screen	▪ Relapse prevention I: Seemingly irrelevant decisions	▪ Anger management
▪ Introductions and agenda setting	▪ Anticipating high-risk situations	
▪ Round robin check-in: review of self-monitoring and homework		
▪ Homework		
Session 11: Problem-Solving		
▪ BAL/drug screen	▪ Review progress	▪ Problem-solving
▪ Introductions and agenda setting	▪ Anticipating high-risk situations	
▪ Round robin check-in: review of self-monitoring and homework		
▪ Homework		

(continued)

Table 2.1. Continued

Routine Interventions: Alcohol/Drug	Alcohol/Drug-Related Interventions	Female-Specific Interventions

Session 12: Relapse Prevention II, Maintenance Planning

▩ BAL/drug screen	▩ Relapse prevention II:	
▩ Introductions and agenda setting	▩ Identifying and managing warning signs of relapse	
▩ Round robin check-in: review of self-monitoring and homework	▩ Handling slips and relapses	
▩ Homework for continuing group members	▩ Relapse contract	
	▩ Farewell to member leaving group	
	▩ High-risk situations	

There is strong empirical support for the effectiveness of CBT approaches to alcohol and drug use and these other problems (Mastroleo & Monti, 2013). High-quality CBT is personalized to each client and guided by an individualized case conceptualization of the development and maintenance of AUD or SUD and related problems. The female-only group format of the treatment lowers barriers to access and provides a supportive, safe environment to directly address substance use and related problems as well as an opportunity to enhance a sober support network for abstinence. This treatment program provides an optimal hybrid of expert guidance through state-of-the-art CBT with the support of other women with shared experiences and challenges to assist one another through the difficult journey of overcoming AUD or SUD and developing a substance-free lifestyle.

Motivational Enhancement

General therapeutic stance

CBT therapists function as content experts and to some degree supportive coaches. They collaborate with and treat each client with respect and as a person of value. Exploring each client's subjective experience, as well as the details of her daily life, is necessary to understand the function of alcohol or drugs in her life. The use of some motivational enhancement therapy strategies and motivational interviewing (MI) techniques (see Miller & Rollnick, 2013) is recommended. For instance, "MI spirit" includes accurate reflective listening (especially in response to clients' substance-related change or commitment talk), empathy, and "rolling with resistance." These are considered basic necessary therapeutic skills and are an integral part of the high-quality CBT described in this Therapist Guide. These therapeutic skills are combined with specific, structured aspects of the therapy. CBT therapists are not confrontational or overly directive, but do provide structure, expert opinion, psychoeducation, and constructive corrective feedback around skills the women are learning. The therapeutic stance is collaborative and supportive.

Assessment feedback

In the first session, the therapist provides feedback to each client about the extent, severity, and consequences of her drinking/drug use. Such feedback has been demonstrated to enhance motivation to change. This is done in the group setting to generate universality of experience among the group members and reciprocal support, as well as to help reduce the shame associated with drinking/drug use and to increase acceptance of the understanding that problematic alcohol and drug use are treatable conditions, not personal failures or flaws.

Decisional balance

In Session 4, the therapist and clients begin a decisional balance exercise, which is revisited throughout treatment. This exercise helps the client be more aware of the decision she has made to change, acknowledges the perceived social or emotional losses associated with stopping drinking or drug use, and highlights reasons to stop using drugs/alcohol (focusing on both the damage that use has wreaked in her life and the positive aspects of overcoming addiction). The decisional balance also allows the therapist and other group members to share their empathy about the difficulty in stopping alcohol/drug use, and highlights the gains the client may realize from abstinence.

Reinforcing abstinence and increasing salience of negative consequences of alcohol/drug use

By developing behavior chains around the antecedents and consequences of her substance use in specific situations (functional analysis), the client learns to link the negative consequences of drinking/drug use in response to each of her triggers. This repeated focus on the reasons to stop and the benefits of not drinking or using drugs reinforces motivation to change and helps to maintain abstinence.

Linking recovery from related problems to benefits of stopping drinking/drug use

In constructing decisional matrices and behavior chains, the therapist should take into account each client's case conceptualization and help her understand how other problems such as depression, avoidance of trauma cues, anxiety, shame, an over-critical internal voice, or other issues might contribute to maintaining her drinking/drug use and how these other issues are likely to be difficult to treat as long as the client continues to drink/use drugs. Knowing that cessation of alcohol/drug use will free them to move on and address other areas of distress may be frightening but also can be a key motivator for women to stop using substances, take ownership of their life direction, resolve other areas of distress, and initiate steps to build a happier and more productive lifestyle.

Alcohol/Drug-Focused Coping Skills

Functional analysis (behavior chains)

The functional analysis is central to individualized CBT planning. Through the behavior chain and related exercises, the therapist and client identify triggers/high-risk situations that place the client at high risk for drinking, as well as the cognitive and affective responses that follow. Therapy then progresses by systematically helping the client learn ways to modify high-risk situations, learn different cognitive responses to the high-risk situations, learn new behaviors to use in response to high-risk situations, use insight about the positive consequences of drinking to learn new ways to obtain similar positive reinforcers through means other than drinking, and learn to focus on the negative consequences of drinking in high-risk situations. The therapist needs to be careful to use terms that clients understand (e.g., "behavior chain" instead of "functional analysis") and also to teach the clients how to use the skill going forward.

Identifying triggers/high-risk situations

This is accomplished through interviewing, developing a triggers list in Session 2, and having the client record triggers on her daily self-recording cards. Worksheets help the client think of triggers in different areas of her life. The therapist can offer suggestions as well—triggers specific to each season, for instance, or subtle triggers the therapist noticed that may be operative in each client's life.

Identifying and coping with unhelpful thoughts

The therapist uses behavior chains to help clients learn about the links among triggers, thoughts, feelings, and behaviors, and in later sessions helps clients learn about the importance of slowing down their thought process to recognize unhelpful thoughts. The therapist also helps the client identify dysfunctional thoughts about herself and others, as well as identifying her positive expectancies about the effects she anticipates from drinking/using drugs. Unhelpful thoughts about alcohol/drugs are also explicitly targeted using cognitive restructuring techniques in Session 8.

Identifying and coping with negative emotions

This also is accomplished primarily through careful interviewing, helping clients differentiate thoughts from feelings, and discussing emotions identified while completing specific behavior chains with the clients in the group. Also, in Sessions 5, 6, 7, and 10, mood and emotion regulation are addressed directly, to help change habitual (but unhelpful) ways of feeling and handling emotions and to reduce acute stress reactivity.

Identifying consequences of drinking/drug use

Consequences are assessed pre-treatment, during completion of specific behavior chains, and in the decisional matrix. The therapist often has to help the client become more aware of the consequences, either positive or negative, of drinking or drug use in specific situations. Using some MI techniques, the therapist tries to elicit and also selectively reinforce reasons to change ("change talk") through the use of simple or complex reflections (Miller & Rollnick, 2013), and selectively responds less to reasons not to change ("sustain talk"), in order to help consolidate the client's beliefs about reasons to stop drinking/using drugs. Also, the therapist helps the client remind herself about the "plus side" of abstinence; research shows that it is the positive consequences of not drinking or using drugs that contribute most strongly to the maintenance of abstinence, so clients must learn to keep those salient by noting and tracking them.

Changing triggers and/or coping with them effectively

From the client's personalized list of triggers, the therapist works with her to plan strategies ("self-management plans") to respond to high-risk environmental triggers without drinking/drug use.

Changing thoughts and feelings

Cognitive therapy interventions targeted to changing unhelpful thoughts and feelings are included in behavior chains, coping with cravings, dealing with alcohol/drug-related thoughts, and, to some degree, the decisional matrix exercise described above under motivational interventions. Feelings are also targeted directly via cognitive therapy techniques in sessions on handling depression, anxiety, trauma, emotion regulation, and anger.

Changing behavior

Clients identify reciprocal relationships among situations, thoughts, feelings, behaviors, and consequences of behaviors, in the service of positive outcomes. Alcohol/drug use behavior change is a primary outcome variable targeted in the program via skills training (drink refusal, self-management planning, etc.) as well as by increasing motivation to stop using substances.

Changing consequences

The functional analysis and decisional matrix help the client become aware of positive consequences she believes she experiences from drinking or drug use and help her identify alternative ways to obtain replacement reinforcers. Making abstinence rewarding is also targeted in the Therapist Guide via overall better quality of life. Clients also practice making negative consequences of substance use more salient.

Dealing with cravings

Session 6 helps clients acquire an understanding of cravings and devise strategies to cope effectively with them.

Relapse prevention

The treatment draws on several of Marlatt and Gordon's (1985) original concepts of relapse prevention. The entire Therapist Guide and companion Client Workbook are, in some respects, a relapse prevention treatment, since every session focuses on identification and anticipation of high-risk situations and use of alternative coping skills. The last part of the treatment focuses more explicitly on relapse prevention and maintenance of positive change after treatment ends, introducing the notion that most clients do slip or relapse, and developing a set of strategies to both avoid relapses and cope with slips/relapses that may occur.

Female-Specific Aspects of the Treatment Program

This treatment program includes several interventions and themes that are highly prevalent among women with AUD/SUD and are also targeted as additional outcomes of treatment.

Core Thematic Women's Issues

Two core therapeutic themes related to women's lives are integrated into the structure and content of the program throughout the 12 sessions. Specific examples, discussion, interventions, and illustrative material are given in the Therapist Guide, guided by these themes:

1. **The woman as an active agent in her own life:** One goal of the female-specific therapy is to create and/or enhance a sense of autonomy and self-confidence for each woman. Therapists work to help each client view herself as a competent person capable of managing her life and creating meaning and happiness for herself. The goal is to help the client feel more self-confident as an effective coper, and to be less emotionally reactive to situations and people around her—to care less what others think about her, especially if her self-value had been primarily based on others' perception of her.

2. **The woman's right to balance self-care versus other-care:** A second goal of the female-specific therapy is to strengthen each woman's belief that she is a lovable person worthy of the respect and love of others, as well as worthy of her own self-respect, self-compassion, and self-care, and that she deserves the same level of attention from herself that she gives to others. The importance and quality of relationships in her life is highlighted but balanced with her ability to take her own needs into account. Likewise, responsibilities in a woman's life should be balanced with self-care and enjoyable activities. This is

both a theme and a content area, with specific interventions to identify and amplify self-care in thoughts and behaviors.

Female-Specific Content: Six Areas of Improved Coping

This program focuses explicitly on six areas to enhance women's coping:

1. Self-care in thoughts (self-compassion vs. shame) and behaviors (healthy lifestyle changes)
2. Coping with anxiety, including cognitive, behavioral, and acceptance-based strategies to recognize types and manifestations of anxiety and anxious thinking, to alleviate anxiety
3. Coping with depression, using cognitive, behavioral, and acceptance-based strategies to recognize clinical depression and depressive thinking and to alleviate depression
4. Understanding and managing trauma symptoms
5. Learning emotion regulation skills and anger management to reduce stress reactivity
6. Improving interpersonal skills and social network support for abstinence, including managing the presence of heavy drinkers in one's social network; connecting with others for healthy, supportive relationships; assertiveness training; and effective communication skills.

Other high-risk situations and drinking antecedents of particular relevance for women with alcohol or drug problems are highlighted in the course of discussing these six topics. Various issues are addressed through the skills training interventions, such as the use of alcohol in response to sexual dysfunction, loneliness, relationships, parenting issues, body image, "sandwich generation" issues (i.e., taking care of elderly parents while also raising children), menopause, role loss, multiple role stress, and physiological triggers such as craving and premenstrual dysphoria.

What Else Is Female-Specific About This Treatment Program?

All group members are women. The female-specific interventions were chosen based on the high incidence of these related problems among female problem drinkers. The group process is used to facilitate discussion of issues that are germane to the women in the group and to create a feeling of "commonality" and support among group members through shared female experiences. All vignettes, sample worksheets, and sample therapist dialogues provided in the Therapist Guide and Client Workbook are female-relevant. Psychoeducational material is provided to educate the clients about the ways in which women uniquely use, process, and suffer from heavy use of alcohol and drugs.

Not all of the clients will have histories of all the problems covered in the Therapist Guide and Client Workbook, but most of the modules are likely to help most women. For instance, not all women experience clinical levels of anxiety and depression; however, many women tend to struggle with anxiety and depression at least occasionally at a sub-clinical level, and all women, even those who experience only fleeting symptoms, will benefit from learning how to identify and manage anxiety and depression. Likewise, in terms of social support networks and heavy drinking or drug use by significant others, not all women will have social support networks that are unsupportive or are conducive to drinking or drug use. However, since women tend to place high value on their social networks, incorporating standard sections into the program to address issues related to social support is likely to be relevant on some level to most female clients.

Gender-neutral CBT groups for SUD typically focus only on alcohol/drug-related interventions. For instance, the treatment may include drink refusal training, but not general assertiveness training. There typically is no explicit intervention related to comorbid disorders or affect management. If, for example, depression is discussed, it is as a trigger for drinking or drug use, not as a treatment target in its own right. There may be a section on dealing with alcohol/drug-related thoughts, but not cognitive restructuring for any other category of thoughts. In contrast, this female-specific program is designed with a broader focus. Rather than content being used solely in the service of teaching alcohol-related skills, it is the other way around: Teaching of alcohol/drug-related skills is presented and taught in the context of women's issues. Dual goals guide the therapy in every session: (a) abstinence from alcohol/drugs and (b) highlighting and discussing women's issues in their own right, in addition to how they relate to alcohol/drug use. In other words, rather than being considered as secondary outcomes, improving outcomes related to issues such as depression, anxiety, social support, autonomy, and self-care are considered to be equally important as the outcome of abstinence from alcohol or drug use.

CHAPTER 3

How to Use This Therapist Guide and Client Workbook

Typical Structure of Sessions

The treatment program we outline in this Therapist Guide is a hybrid of interpersonal support, group process, and structured skills training. The treatment combines didactic presentations of coping skills, motivational material, group discussion, and skills rehearsal with an interactive environment providing mutual emotional support and support for change efforts. As the therapist, you will use a motivational enhancement approach and nonspecific factors from motivational interviewing (MI) to facilitate change, and introduce coping skills in a collaborative, non-confrontational way. Each session is structured similarly: (a) welcome; (b) review of the session agenda; (c) round robin check-in regarding self-monitoring of drinking/drug use, cravings, triggers, and homework; (d) introduction of new skills using handouts and sample worksheets; (e) practice of new skills in group; (f) plan for upcoming high-risk situations; and (g) assignment of homework.

Client Workbook

Before her first session each client should obtain a Client Workbook, which includes all the handouts and worksheets she will need for the sessions. It is helpful to provide a link to a site where clients can purchase the workbook; alternatively, you could provide each client with a workbook at the assessment or her first session and roll the cost of the workbook into the first session fee. Note that all handouts and worksheets appear both in this Therapist Guide and in the companion Client Workbook; to facilitate use of the workbook, the guide includes workbook page cross-references for every handout and worksheet—for example, "Handout 1.1: Treatment Contract appears in Client Workbook page."

The weekly handouts include informational sheets that reiterate and expand on material covered in session, sample skills-training worksheets, and blank worksheets used to learn and practice the skills. Group members use their workbooks during and between sessions to master skills, and as a tool to help prevent relapse after treatment ends.

"Round Robin" Interventions and Modeling

For routine interventions such as a check-in about substance use and cravings for the prior week, and planning for high-risk situations, a "round robin" method (Sobell & Sobell, 2011) is used. For check-in about substance use/cravings, for instance, the therapist goes around the room and asks each woman to give a brief description of how her week went in terms of drinking and drug use triggers and cravings while the therapist follows along, reviewing the client's daily self-monitoring logs. You may ask about days on which there was a slip, or a trigger with no slip, or intense cravings. Group members listen to each other and provide support, encouragement, and constructive ideas about how triggers/cravings might have been dealt with differently. Group member comments to other members such as, "Oh, it was okay to drink because you really had a rough week" or "You've been really good; you deserved to have a drink this week," should be discouraged by redirecting the conversation to the rest of the group with a question like, "Yes, that was a tough week. Do others have any thoughts about what xxx could have done differently in this situation to avoid drinking or using drugs that day?" Feedback from the assessment and planning for high-risk situations each week similarly uses the round robin format.

As the therapist, you will introduce a new skill in each session; modeling and practice with the new skill is accomplished with group volunteers and group participation. For each new skill, you will model use of the skill with a group member volunteer as the other women watch and follow along while providing input and support to the volunteer and also filling in their own worksheets for the skill.

When you introduce new content or practice the skills with the group or a specific volunteer, you should use a flipchart or whiteboard/chalkboard to introduce the topic and rationale for each new coping skill and to facilitate practicing the new skill. As the therapist, you should actively write on the flipchart while walking through a worksheet with a volunteer. For instance, you might draw the four empty cells of the decisional matrix worksheet on the flipchart and write in the volunteer's responses in each cell. Encourage group members to bring their workbooks to group each week and to complete their own worksheets for each topic during the session. We have found that when women complete worksheets during the group session, they are more likely to use the skill and remember helpful tips from other members. Use only one group volunteer at a time to demonstrate most skills, to show clearly how the skill can be applied meaningfully to a group member's substance use pattern in the context of her day-to-day life. Once you complete the skill demonstration with the volunteer, the group can ask questions, give feedback, and relate the topic to their own situations.

Individual Treatment Adaptation

The Therapist Guide and Client Workbook are written for use in a therapy group, the most common modality for community addiction treatment (Roman, 2013). However, this Therapist Guide is identical, except for the group components, to an individual alcohol use disorder (AUD) treatment manual for female-specific cognitive behavioral therapy (CBT) that we developed and tested prior to creating the group version (Epstein et al., 2018b). To deliver this treatment in individual therapy, the therapist may simply use the Therapist Guide and leave out any material relevant for group delivery; otherwise, the content is the same. The companion Client Workbook can also be used in either group or individual treatment.

Using a Structured Treatment Guide in a Clinically Meaningful Way

Treatment is not meant to be delivered in either a "cookie cutter" or lecture style. Follow the Therapist Guide, but integrate your clinical conceptualization of each client with the skills taught in the session. The authors of the Therapist Guide have created substance use disorder (SUD) treatment interventions and tailored them for women over the course of 30 years; the interventions, sample therapist–client dialogues, vignettes, and example worksheets are relevant to a majority of women with AUD/SUD. Thus, therapists typically find it easy to link the material in the Therapist Guide and Client Workbook to specific women's AUD/SUD experiences, alcohol and other substance use patterns and consequences, and case conceptualizations.

The structure of the sessions lends itself to personalization of the material. Each session starts with a personalized check-in to discuss each client's week in terms of alcohol and other substance use, cravings, coping, challenges, successes, and general well-being. Homework from the prior week is reviewed and discussed. The application of session material takes place in each woman's daily life, and the homework is designed to link new coping skills introduced during the group with between-session application. After the initial review of the week and homework, a new topic is introduced along with a rationale linking the topic to each specific client's ongoing concerns and challenges. In session, you and the group members will review worksheet examples that illustrate how the material might be applied to a typical female-specific situation. These examples both clarify how the specific coping skill is used in a clinically meaningful way, and universalize and normalize the struggles of women with SUD. Over the years we have regularly had clients exclaim, "That's me! I do exactly that!" when reading over a sample completed worksheet. A blank worksheet for the session's coping skill is then completed collaboratively in group to apply the coping skills to each woman's personal situation. If the worksheets are not finished in session, the women complete the worksheet for homework (practice assignment) that week, and are encouraged to try out the skill during the week as well. Thus, the practice exercises individualize and personalize every topic and skill covered in the Therapist Guide.

The topics introduced in each session are meant to be repetitive and cumulative. As treatment progresses clients are taught to incorporate each skill into an accumulating coping skills toolkit to use as needed, and to continue practicing all new and previous skills each week.

Outpatient Versus Inpatient Versus Aftercare

This program can be used as a stand-alone outpatient treatment in a community outpatient clinic or private practice, or can be used as a weekly group as part of a more intensive ambulatory treatment setting such as an intensive outpatient program (IOP). It also can be used as part of the treatment program in an SUD treatment setting, either in full or by delivering specific sessions; in detoxification units (for instance, Session 1) or as part of inpatient rehabilitation programming; or as a coping skills group in a residential non-treatment setting such as a women's sober house.

Some parts of the treatment will be more relevant to one setting than another. For example, in outpatient treatment women may still be drinking or using drugs and want to stop. In that setting, decision-making around detoxification and development of abstinence plans will be important. In contrast, for aftercare settings women typically will already be abstinent, so the focus on detoxification and abstinence plans will be less relevant. In addition, in aftercare settings (e.g., a post-inpatient IOP or a sober house), the assessment will be more limited (see Chapter 5 for details) and the assessment feedback can be briefer.

Inpatient and aftercare settings also may require other adaptations of the treatment. If participants do not need the skills to stop drinking or using drugs, the same skills may be framed as relapse prevention. For example, the women may be helped to identify drinking/drug use triggers from before treatment, and identify new triggers they are experiencing now or anticipate upon returning home (also note that that each new season of the year typically has a unique set of triggers). Other skills also may be framed as relapse prevention so that clients leave treatment prepared to deal with high-risk situations. The women-specific interventions that do not focus specifically on alcohol or drugs are used the same way regardless of setting or population.

Alcohol Versus Other Drug Use

The treatment guide can be applied to AUD or other SUDs. The session process, content, and skills introduced in this therapy are equally applicable to different substances that women in the group may be using. It is important to educate yourself about the differences in use patterns, methods of administration, effects, withdrawal symptoms, and doses of any drug that the client is using. (See the National Institute of Drug Abuse website [https://nida.nih.gov/] for detailed information on every drug of abuse.) Your detailed knowledge about specific drugs will come in handy to help the client personalize triggers and understand cravings and consequences of use of each specific drug. For instance, substances differ from one another in patterns of use and the risk profile of withdrawal syndromes, so a thorough understanding of use patterns and withdrawal profiles for each substance is necessary to help clients develop safe and relevant abstinence plans, and to construct relevant behavior chains.

In our studies, the modal use pattern for alcohol among women with AUD was one or two bottles (five to 10 standard drinks) of wine per evening (a steady, daily drinking pattern), often alone, or sometimes starting with a glass of wine while cooking or eating dinner but then continuing to drink in secret after the meal. Wine was the most common type of alcohol consumed among the women in our research, followed by vodka and then beer. In contrast, cocaine typically is used in a binge pattern, rather than daily. Benzodiazepines are extremely addictive, they typically are used in a daily pattern, and the withdrawal profile is dangerous; like alcohol, it can potentially be fatal, and can also include psychosis, among other symptoms. Opiates also are usually used daily, and cessation of use typically is followed by a period of intensely uncomfortable withdrawal that many clients may attempt to manage on their own using stockpiled or "street-purchased" suboxone. Drinking and drug use patterns and preferences differ by culture, age group, family constellation, and sexual orientation.

The language and terminology specific to alcohol versus other substances differ. Generally, saying "intoxicated" for alcohol and "high" for drugs is one simple way to handle this. Methods to obtain illicit substances (compared to alcohol) often are more marginalized, creating substance-specific negative consequences such as illegal activities to pay for and obtain the drugs. Another clinical issue derives from the psychoactive effects of different substances. Group members whose primary substance is alcohol may not relate to the psychoactive effects or consequences of stimulants (such as cocaine or methamphetamines) or the perception-altering effects of hallucinogenic drugs. For each of these issues, the challenge is to help group members share their unique experiences and to help group members find commonality in these experiences and empathy for each other's struggles regardless of the specific substance they are using. Discourage critical, confrontational, or judgmental interactions among group members, and encourage empathy and support.

Clients with Non-Abstinence Goals

The Therapist Guide and Client Workbook focus on skills to achieve and maintain abstinence from the current problem substance. Abstinence is generally not a controversial goal for drugs other than cannabis. In contrast, many clients are ambivalent about setting an abstinence goal for alcohol. The Therapist Guide provides a rationale and discussion of reasons to be abstinent at least for the duration of the treatment protocol (see Chapter 4). In discussing goals, be aware that alcohol is a common trigger for cocaine and other drug use, so typically drug treatment programs expect cessation of alcohol as well; similarly, use of cannabis and other drugs can be a trigger for drinking, so it is generally advisable to address this when constructing the triggers list for each client and recommending abstinence accordingly. However, if you wish to use this Therapist Guide for clients with a moderation goal, most of the interventions can be adapted by adding additional psychoeducation on risky versus non-risky drinking and modifying the interventions to accommodate a moderation goal. We do not, however, recommend mixing clients with abstinence goals in a group with clients with moderation goals.

There is the potential for tensions among group members depending on their change goals around alcohol and other substances. A woman dependent on alcohol may use marijuana occasionally (and live in a state where the drug is legal); a woman whose primary problem substance is marijuana may have an occasional glass of wine without negative consequences. The treatment program focuses on abstinence from the substance causing problems to each woman, and addresses use of other substances in an individualized way. We have, however, found in one pilot study that women who continued to use other drugs during our group or individual AUD treatment had worse AUD outcomes. Thus, we typically advise women to try abstinence from all substances at least during the 12-week course of the group therapy. Women and providers in many treatment settings who accept a 12-step model of addiction have strong opinions about the need for complete abstinence from all substances. Regardless, helping group members respect and accept differences in goals is a challenge; allowing the women to discuss these differences in group in a reasoned and supportive way can be helpful to motivate change in unhealthy behaviors.

Closed Versus Rolling-Admission Groups

Closed Groups

Therapy groups can be "closed"—that is, a group begins with all members starting together at Session 1 and continues through 12 sessions together. No new members enter the group after Session 1. A closed group allows for stronger and more meaningful social support connections among the members and facilitates a step-by-step progression through the treatment program. The sessions build on one another as all members are at the same or similar stages of recovery at each session. However, a closed group format is difficult to execute in private practice and community treatment settings as it requires amassing six to eight women to begin at the same time, and due to attrition, the group size may dwindle to very few women. Closed groups are most feasible in an environment where there is a large and steady flow of women who seek treatment for AUD, with several closed groups starting each week or two so that a wait to begin a new group would not be longer than 2 to 3 weeks.

Assessment prior to joining closed group

Before joining the group, each woman should have an individual assessment session (see Chapter 5) to determine the appropriate level of her initial care and to evaluate her suitability for the group. Assessment is also necessary to gather information on pre-treatment patterns of alcohol/drug use, as well other treatment needs that are integrated into the group Session 1 assessment/feedback intervention. For closed groups, the therapist or clinic would provide the assessment session a week or two prior to group Session 1, and for all the members, assessment/feedback interventions occur in Session 1.

Open Rolling-Admission Groups

In most clinical settings, "open" ("rolling admission") treatment groups are provided to allow for timely entry into an ongoing group, and to maintain a group membership of six to eight women at any time. If an open group gets too big, additional open groups can be started and run concurrently. For an open group, each session has to be stand-alone in that material cannot build systematically on prior sessions as in a closed group, since new clients are joining at any group. Once a client attends all 12 sessions—based on available space and the needs of the client and clinical setting—the client could continue in the same open group for additional sessions for ongoing support or additional practice with the skills. Or, clients could be allowed to attend only 12 sessions to maintain space for new clients. Therapists and clinics can flexibly design the women-specific group structure as necessary. For instance, a "train station" model can be used, such that the group begins as a closed group with at least three members, and then additional cohorts of women can enter the group at Sessions 4 and 8, so that only three of 12 group sessions will need to include ways to introduce and incorporate new members.

Assessment prior to joining a rolling-admission group

For rolling-admission groups, each new member should have an individual assessment (see above for closed group, and also see Chapter 5) with the group facilitator prior to joining the group.

Brief orientation to group for women joining rolling-admission group after Session 1

At the end of the assessment session, for women joining the group at any session (i.e., Session 2–12) after Session 1, the therapist should spend an additional 30 minutes with each woman to provide a brief session orientation in which the therapist provides the Client Workbook and also reviews basic information covered in Session 1 that the client will need to know in order to proceed with all subsequent sessions. This information includes how to use the Client Workbook; group rules; and a brief review of core treatment elements, including self-monitoring, psychoeducation, high-risk situations, triggers, and behavior chains (see Session 2). That way, no matter what session the new member is entering, she will be able to do daily self-monitoring and understand the basics of high-risk situations, triggers, and behavior chains.

Introducing incoming members in rolling-admission group

Each rolling-admission group session with a new member starts with a 5-minute introduction and a 10-minute assessment feedback to the new member. Members in the group at different stages of recovery can provide support to the new client, and share their own feedback from their first session. If a new member is lacking relevant information from previous sessions, she can review sessions in the workbook or you can briefly describe the section, and/or abstinent members can be encouraged to spend time with the new member after session to explain relevant prior material.

Optional graphing intervention for outpatient treatment settings

Graphing group members' drinking/drug use and urge data (from their self-monitoring cards) is an optional intervention that therapists may or may not choose to include as part of the treatment. In closed groups, this optional graphing section would be introduced in Session 2, and in open rolling-admission groups, it would be introduced to each new woman at the session after her first week of completing daily monitoring cards. In sessions after the optional graphing intervention is introduced, the client or therapist updates the graph with summarized weekly data from the daily monitoring cards.

In the pre-session sign-in, using pre-treatment information from the assessment, start a graph (see Handout 2.1: Graph: Alcohol/Drug Use and Urges Sample and Worksheet 2.1: Graph: Alcohol/Drug Use and Urges) for each woman in the group (or for one woman in individual therapy). Enter each woman's pre-treatment average number of standard drinks per week and average number of drug use days per week from before treatment. During check-in, you will help each woman enter the pre-treatment information before her first session, and then at each session during the check-in you will help each woman enter her weekly drinking, drug use, and cravings data into her graph in her workbook. Or, if you prefer, you can start each client's graph with the pre-treatment information, update each client's weekly graph during the individual check-in, and give the updated graph to each woman to use and discuss during the group. (You can print an updated graph for each woman each week if you use a spreadsheet to enter the daily monitoring data each week, or you can update a handwritten graph manually.)

Each group member should look at her updated graph: the x-axis is time (the baseline and 12 sessions) and the y-axis has up to four data points:

1. Total number of standard drinks consumed for the week (for women who are drinking)
2. Number of days used a drug (for women who are using a drug)
3. Total number of urges during the week (urge frequency for alcohol and/or drugs)
4. Average strength of urges during the week (on a scale of 1–7).

When you start each woman's graph, you will also be creating the y-axis for each graph tailored to the upper limit of standard drinks (based on pre-treatment assessment) and the drugs each woman reported using at baseline. Urges strength will correspond to a scale of 1 to 7 toward the bottom of the y-axis. Generally, a y-axis of 0 to 50 or 60 in increments of 2 or 5 is typical, but it will vary across group members.

Explain to the group that graphing the data each week will help them track their progress.

Note that we use the terms "urge" (to use) and "craving" interchangeably—they mean the same thing.

This treatment program can be used in conjunction with other outpatient individual, couple, and/or family therapy. The treatment also is compatible with concurrent pharmacotherapy for detoxification, alcohol cravings (e.g., naltrexone, injectable naltrexone, acamprosate, topiramate, gabapentin, or baclofen), alcohol aversion medication (disulfiram), or other medication-assisted therapies (MAT) such as suboxone or methadone. It also is compatible with medications for co-morbid psychiatric problems often seen in populations of women with AUD/SUD, such as depression, anxiety, post-traumatic stress disorder, and bipolar disorder. The treatment approach is generally not compatible with medications that induce physiological dependence, such as benzodiazepines, opiates, barbiturates, or stimulants, and we generally discourage use of addictive or habit-forming sleep aids. Cross-tolerance may be likely for clients with SUD, and vulnerability to one type of SUD may suggest a heightened vulnerability to other SUDs. These addictive medications also typically have adverse interactions with alcohol and other drugs, and may put the client at risk for developing another addiction, even if used as prescribed.

Therapists are encouraged to obtain consents to communicate with each woman's other providers and to consult/collaborate with providers about specific cases. It is common for us to recommend a psychiatric consultation for AUD or SUD medications, and/or for other co-morbid psychiatric problems. Consultation with specialists in addiction medicine is preferred so that the woman will not be prescribed medications that might worsen current SUD and/or create a new addiction. Collaboration with other providers (e.g., primary care physicians, other therapists, recovery coaches) is also important. Mutual help groups (e.g., women's Alcoholics Anonymous [AA] groups, Women for Sobriety, Refuge Recovery, yoga recovery groups, SMART Recovery) may be recommended for concurrent support and involvement. It is often helpful to discuss and find commonalities in group members' experiences with mutual help groups, as many strategies and approaches in peer-support groups overlap considerably with our CBT approach but use different language and labels.

This treatment requires that practitioners are knowledgeable about AUD and other SUDs, the unique issues that women with alcohol and drug problems experience, CBT approaches, principles of group therapy, and the unique challenges of therapeutic relationships in group therapy. Given that most practitioners are not experts in all of these areas, this Therapist Guide is structured to facilitate learning how to deliver the program. We have structured the guide to include introductory information about AUD and other SUDs, women's issues, the basics of CBT, and detailed guidance about how to use the Therapist Guide. Each therapy session includes suggested language for the therapist to use to introduce program content and exercises, and potential issues that may arise in the course of group sessions. Chapter 4 describes challenging clinical situations and provides guidance.

To learn the treatment, first read the entire Therapist Guide, including the introductory chapters, so that you'll have a clear understanding of the flow and content of the treatment sessions. In areas where you have less knowledge or experience, additional readings and/or structured trainings would be helpful. However, even for therapists who are experienced in AUD/SUD treatment, working with women and with group therapy involves a learning curve to implement a new treatment program. We suggest the following for successful treatment:

- Keep the Therapist Guide with you and refer to it during the group sessions; it is not expected that you will memorize the guide. Over time the session guides will become familiar enough that the treatment can be delivered mostly just using the handouts/worksheets with a copy of the session agenda.
- Clients should be told to bring their workbook to every group. Have two or three copies of the worksheets for the session in case a client forgets her workbook.
- Thoroughly review the session materials prior to each group so you can tailor the session material to the clients in the group.
- Review abstinence plans and homework (including the self-monitoring cards) thoroughly at each session. The value of homework assignments in CBT cannot be understated. Reviewing homework assignments each session conveys their importance and

also reinforces skill acquisition. If some clients are not completing the homework, reinforce its importance and problem-solve barriers to completing homework.

- Each session presents particular and essential skills. For instance, a client can take the group off on a tangent that could derail the focus on skills. We have found that client and group tangents usually can be tied back to the session content.

- Use the power of the group whenever possible. Group members can give each other feedback and model successful change efforts. They also can help an individual group member get back on track if she is on a tangent.

- Provide a clear rationale for the skills presented in each session. Be sure to review the rationale for each skill slowly and thoroughly, and check in with the group to make sure they understand the rationale.

CHAPTER 4

Clinical and Group Management Issues in Women's CBT Group for SUD

Ambivalence About Change

Every therapist working with women (and men) with alcohol use disorder (AUD) or other substance use disorders (SUDs) is familiar with clients' mixed feelings about changing or continuing to drink or use drugs. Reasons not to change are myriad—habit and the familiarity of using, physiological or psychological dependence, psychological needs that the substance meets, the social context that supports use, fear of the unknown, lack of skills, and lack of support for change are only a few of the reasons that clients talk about. But something drives them to seek treatment, typically the negative consequences of use that have become intolerable, external pressures to change, a vision of a better or different life, and/or concern about feeling out of control of the use (Grosso et al., 2013). When women start treatment, they usually are focused on the negative consequences they would like to eliminate and often lack a vision of an alternative, more positive life without alcohol or drugs. This ambivalence plays out in a woman's language about alcohol and drugs or about changes, with "sustain" talk for continued use counterbalanced by "change" talk for stopping her alcohol or drug use (see Session 4). Ambivalence also plays out in women's behavior, and may be seen in their continued substance use, not completing between-session assignments, and/or coming late to or missing group sessions. Miller and Rollnick (2013) provide more detail about and clinical techniques for addressing ambivalence and motivation. Women's CBT Group for SUD draws upon motivational interviewing (MI) spirit (see Chapter 3) as one way to address ambivalence. You do not need to learn MI to use this treatment program, but you should become familiar with ways to listen for, selectively reinforce, and elicit client "change talk" (which we think of as a proxy for client "change think"). Some women express "sustain talk" (which reflects "sustain think") because they lack the skills to effect change and do not have a vision for what change would even look like. Our treatment model assumes that some early successes with behavior change will increase the woman's motivation to continue to change and decrease her motivation to continue to use. Thus, taking action by working on cognitive behavioral therapy (CBT) skills that facilitate change should increase women's self-efficacy for coping with their alcohol or drug use. Initial behavior change typically leads to some positive results, which enhance motivation for further change.

Goal Setting and Getting There: Abstinence Versus Moderation

At the initial intake the therapist will talk with each woman about her substance use goals and let the woman know that the treatment focuses on abstinence as the least risky alternative to her present alcohol or drug use. This discussion of goals does not focus on life-long abstinence, but rather focuses on abstinence during the treatment to give her an opportunity to get experience with being abstinent and developing skills to maintain change. If the woman is unwilling to make a commitment to at least strive for abstinence during the 3-month treatment period, the group setting may not be clinically indicated for her. We do not expect clients to become abstinent immediately. Rather, we work with each client to create an abstinence plan starting in Session 1 if they are still using. The treatment program is geared toward achieving abstinence by the fifth therapy session, but sooner quit dates are preferable if safe.

If a client's stated goal is some form of moderation, ask the client specifics about what frequency/quantity of drinking/drug use she has in mind when she says "moderation." Amounts for drinking can be compared to National Institute on Alcohol Abuse and Alcoholism (NIAAA) limits for low-risk drinking for women: no more than seven standard drinks per week and no more than one standard drink on any day. (NIAAA defines heavy drinking as more than three standard drinks in a day for women.) Often clients' views of moderation are distorted and above such limits. It is usually helpful to share, in a collaborative and non-judgmental way, our rationale for asking clients to consider choosing an abstinence goal for the term of the treatment:

I noticed on your form that you indicated that your ideal goal would be to reduce your drinking/drug use, or to use occasionally. Our group is designed to help women stop drinking/using drugs completely during treatment. Would you be willing to commit yourself to work toward becoming abstinent during the 3-month treatment?

If, after discussion, the woman does not want to commit to trying abstinence during the treatment period, the group is probably not appropriate for her. You should provide other treatment options to such clients to support their desire to change their drinking or drug use, and a treatment that is congruent with their goals is likely to help them reduce their use and therefore reduce their risk for adverse consequences of continuing to use at their current, risky level.

If the woman appears ambivalent about abstinence or is unclear about the rationale for abstinence, there are several ways for you to address this ambivalence:

1. Acknowledge that ambivalence is common.
2. Explain that the program emphasizes abstinence during treatment to give the client an opportunity to learn more about the role of drinking/drug use in her life and learn alternative coping skills, and that by the end of the treatment the woman will have more information and experience to help her think through her future goals.
3. Note the value of abstinence in terms of safety and health.
4. Discuss the difference between "controlled" drinking, which requires careful monitoring and self-vigilance, and "social" drinking, which is drinking occasionally without issues or need for self-control.
5. Note contraindications to "controlled" drinking for women with significant medical or psychiatric problems or a family history of AUD.
6. Note that "controlled" drug use has not been studied among persons with SUD and is not recommended.

This can be a difficult conversation. Since it is extremely common for women to begin treatment with a preference to cut back but not stop drinking, we provide a sample way to express the notion of trying abstinence while in the women's group:

It's very common for people who come to treatment for alcohol (and some- times cannabis) problems to say that they would like to have a drink now and then, or do "controlled drinking" (or "social drinking," also called "moderated drinking"). Our program is abstinence-based, and while we don't ask you to commit to remaining abstinent your whole life, we do ask that you make a commitment to try to become and stay abstinent during the 3 months you're in treatment with us. Why? First, we want you to have a stretch of time with alcohol/drugs out of your life, so that you can get used to it a bit, and see what it's like. Often people don't realize how much alcohol/drugs play a role in their lives until the substance use is gone for a while.

Second, we want to give you skills to be abstinent and have you practice them over the next 3 months, so that you will always have those skills should you want to use them.

The third reason is that abstinence is always the safest choice. You won't have alcohol- or drug-related problems if you're not drinking/using drugs. And it's a very common relapse pattern to start out with "just one drink/drug" here and there, and then slide the slippery slope to problem drinking or drug use over time.

Fourth, controlled or moderated drinking is not the same as social drinking. Social drinkers can have a drink once a week or less, but they don't really think about drinking otherwise—they can take it or leave it. Controlled (or moderated) drinking means continuing to keep alcohol in your life, but constantly working to control it, count drinks, not lose self- control, etc. For many people, it seems that abstinence is easier in the long run than controlled (moderated) drinking, which requires a different focus in treatment.

Fifth, moderated drinking is not usually successful for women with a his- tory of more severe drinking problems and/or a strong genetic vulnerability to alcohol use problems. Regarding drug use, cannabis tends to follow the same rules as drinking—occasional cannabis use may be difficult for people who have had a history of problem use or a strong genetic vulnerability. Drugs like opioids, methamphetamine, amphetamine, benzodiazepines, barbiturates, and nicotine have very high addiction potential, and the negative consequences of any use make these drugs poor candidates for moderated use; abstinence is generally the best and safest choice.

*What are your thoughts? [Discuss client's concerns/response.] After 3 months in this group you can evaluate the pros and cons of abstinence with a clear head and some abstinence experience under your belt, and decide at that point whether you just want to stay abstinent. If you do slip and/or engage in continued use of alcohol or drugs during the 3-month treatment period, we will **not** ask you to leave the group unless we believe you need a higher level of care (and then you will be welcome to join again after). We would work closely with you to use our CBT principles to reverse or minimize slips. If you are strongly considering abstinence and making efforts toward a quit date, we typically will not discharge you from the group.*

If the client asks, "So I can't have a drink for the rest of my life?" or states, "I can't imagine not drinking again for the rest of my life" (or similar remarks), you may respond:

I know that for many people that's one of the hardest thoughts to deal with. I would suggest that you focus on giving yourself a chance to have a chunk of abstinent time so that you can get used to it and find out what it's like. After a 3-month period of abstinence you'll be in a better position to evaluate what it might be like to not drink again. You'll see: You may find that you like life better without alcohol in it.

Continued Drinking/Drug Use

Some women continue to drink or use drugs during treatment. It is important to address this issue until both the client and you understand why it is still occurring. In this treatment model we do NOT discharge clients who are not abstinent or who have slipped or relapsed. We believe that would be akin to not treating a cancer patient for recurring cancer, or discharging a diabetes patient because she is struggling with adherence to her diet. We believe that if clients struggling with changing their drinking/drug use could stop on their own without slipping in the process, they wouldn't be here. We do not condone or reassure clients that slips or continued use are okay, but we do not judge. We also do not use confrontational and/or demotivating statements heard in some treatment programs such as, "Come back when you're ready to stop drinking/using drugs," "Come back when you are ready to stop being resistant," "You have to hit bottom before you will finally stop drinking/drugging," or "You need to stop drinking/drug use for yourself, nobody else." Instead, we assess reasons for the continued use or a slip and try to determine if it is a deficit in motivation, coping skills; strong physical dependence, lack of social supports, and/or comorbid psychopathology that needs to be addressed and then choose an intervention approach accordingly. If it is due to a coping skills problem, we treat continued use or slips matter-of-factly as a problem to analyze by using behavior chains to identify ongoing antecedents and maintaining factors, and then we problem-solve for strategies to try going forward (including possibly recommending a consult with an addiction psychiatrist to add or adjust an anti-craving medication, or an aversion medication [i.e., Antabuse]). Slips and struggles to stop drinking are treated in a compassionate manner, as a behavior that the client can try different ways (and maybe harder) to change, not as a personal flaw or failure.

At each session, review each group member's abstinence plan for clients who are still drinking or using drugs and revise it if some women are not making progress toward their quit date. Some of the most common reasons women continue to use are listed here, with suggested interventions in italics:

1. The woman is struggling with the chosen abstinence plan and is unable to follow it despite her genuine efforts. *It may be time to consider a stronger recommendation for an addiction medicine consult to consider an anti-craving or aversion medication, or, if very little improvement in drinking/drug use has occurred, the need for a higher level of care such as an intensive outpatient program or inpatient treatment, or a detoxification program. The client would be able to resume the group therapy after inpatient care.*

2. The woman no longer wants to strive for complete abstinence. *The client should continue in the group; help her and the group discuss her revised goals using an MI rather than a confrontational style. It is possible that clients will change their drinking goals more than once during treatment and feedback from group members may influence the woman's thinking. Also revisit the decisional matrix or use MI to help the client remember the negative consequences of drinking/drug use that led her to seek treatment and to shift her focus to positive consequences of not using.*

3. The client voices a commitment to abstinence but continues to drink or use at reduced levels. *Determine if the problem is ambivalence and/or coping skills deficits using the Readiness/Confidence Rulers (see* Chapter 5*). If motivation is the problem, use MI spirit skills or revisit the decisional matrix. If continued use is rooted in specific skills deficits or social/environmental challenges, revisit the functional analysis (see Session 2) to help identify specific situations and cognitive and/ or affective variables the client is finding particularly difficult, such as having a sense of helplessness about coping with environmental or internal triggers, attributing responsibility to others, or minimizing the extent or severity of the consequences she experienced from her use.*

If the client is continuing to use alcohol or drugs and also is not completing homework, not attending group regularly, and/or not attempting to implement the skills in response to triggers/cravings during the week, we discuss perceived obstacles to those skills, and attempt to discern whether it is a lack of motivation or skills deficits that needs to be addressed. If repeated attempts fail, we suggest considering the addition of a higher level of care (such as intensive outpatient treatment) to weekly group attendance, or perhaps inpatient detoxification followed by a return to the group.

Suggested interventions for clients who continue to drink/use include:

1. Assess the client's motivation for abstinence; revisit her reasons for seeking treatment and the decisional matrix.
2. Remind the client that this is an abstinence-based treatment program.
3. Identify the situations in which the client is drinking/using drugs.
4. Identify what is getting in the way of quitting (is it a lack of motivation, coping skills deficits, comorbid psychopathology, a desire to switch to a moderation goal, or any combination of these?).
5. Discuss and attempt to resolve obstacles. Discuss the rationale for abstinence during treatment. Help the client choose a target quit date and problem-solve how she can wind down her use.
6. Help the client identify what she could do to get ready for the target quit date.
7. Assess the woman's level of physical dependence and inability to stop without medical supervision. Does the client need a medical detoxification, after which she will return to the group?

Many of our clients show signs of an Axis I disorder (mood, anxiety, eating disorders, etc.). It is important for therapists to be familiar with criteria for Axis I clinical syndromes in the *Diagnostic and Statistical Manual of Mental Disorders* (American Psychiatric Association, 2013) to assess the severity of the problem and refer the client for additional treatment if necessary. You will already have a profile of psychological symptoms from the pre-treatment assessment (see Chapter 5). When assessing the severity of a clinical disorder, you should consider:

1. Suicidality—thoughts, means, plans, history of attempts. If the client presents as an acute suicide risk, you may call the police to have them come to transport the client to a local emergency room.
2. Relationship between drinking and drug use, withdrawal, and psychological symptoms—Withdrawal symptoms may mimic depression and anxiety, in which case they will diminish after a week or two of sobriety, but a woman also may be suffering from a separate anxiety and/or depression disorder that needs treatment. The therapist should monitor the level of depression and anxiety over the course of treatment to evaluate whether the symptoms require separate treatment. In particular, if the pre-treatment assessment suggests a history of comorbid clinical disorders or if symptoms of such disorders develop during treatment, it would be appropriate to refer the woman to an addiction psychiatrist for evaluation, or to a clinician with expertise in evidence-based psychological treatment for the disorder for separate individual therapy.

Many women with AUD or SUD also meet criteria for a personality disorder, with borderline personality, histrionic, and avoidant disorders most common. Individuals with personality disorders may not see the need for their behavior to change and may not be receptive to referrals for additional treatment. It is important that you maintain a clear structure and consistent adherence to boundaries when working with individuals with personality disorders. Use clinical supervision or consultation to get feedback on using various interventions as well as to discuss your own reactions to working with individuals with personality disorders.

Intimate Partner Violence

If intimate partner violence (IPV) is present for any client, assess its current severity/frequency and make a referral for additional treatment if necessary. Some women may believe that they deserve the IPV, may feel guilty about the IPV, or may believe they have no alternatives. Feedback from other women in the group may be beneficial in helping women who feel like this to recognize the importance of taking care of themselves and not accepting violence. In addition to the group discussion and feedback, though, you should consider working with such clients to develop a safety plan (see Epstein et al., 2015).

Parenting

Issues related to parenting commonly come up in women's group sessions. Sometimes challenges with children serve as triggers for alcohol/drug use or urges to use. The group can be helpful in expressing empathy and sharing some common perspectives or experiences and coping strategies. You can guide the discussion to help the client learn how to apply other skills she is learning in the group (e.g., self-management planning, coping with negative emotions) to particular situations with her children. Women also may express guilt and remorse when they believe their use has interfered with their ability to be good parents; skills such as challenging negative thoughts may be helpful here. It may also be helpful to provide referrals to online or community-based parenting skills classes or groups.

If child abuse or neglect is suspected, you may need to assess the situation further in a separate individual meeting. Therapists are legally bound to report cases of suspected child abuse or neglect. If the situation is unclear, consult with a colleague. In some states, child protective services will provide feedback to a therapist about the necessity to report a specific situation (without the therapist sharing any identifying information about the client). Ideally, discuss the situation with the client to inform her that therapists are legally obligated to report suspected child abuse or neglect to child protective services and that the first steps the protective services agency will take will be to open an investigation. It is important to let the client know that your goal is to work with her to ensure that her children are safe. Therapists should follow their organization's policy.

Arriving to Group Intoxicated or High

We recommend administering a breathalyzer or saliva strip for alcohol (and if drugs are a problem for a client, a saliva strip or urine drug screen) during check-in before each group session. If a client registers a positive blood alcohol level (BAL) or appears high or intoxicated, she should not be allowed to attend group that day. There may be instances when the client has a positive alcohol screen but adamantly denies drinking. Almost nothing but alcohol will result in an actual blood alcohol level of .01 or more, although if she had smoked a cigarette just prior to entering the building or had *just* used mouthwash, she could have a spurious reading. When this occurs, wait 10 minutes and then re-administer the alcohol test.

It is important to avoid engaging the client in confrontational interchanges around whether or not she drank. If her second BAL continues to be positive, you can simply inform her that the policy is that she cannot attend group that day. If her BAL is above the legal limit for driving under the influence, she will need to make arrangements to get home safely without operating a vehicle. If her BAL is high enough to potentially be dangerous and she may need medical attention, the safest option is to call 911 or have her call a friend or family member to come pick her up and take her to the nearest emergency room.

Positive drug tests are somewhat more complicated to handle because most drug use yields positive tests several days after last use. If a woman has a positive drug test, determine whether she shows signs of intoxication that would preclude her ability to participate in the group, and also use the test results as information that she is still using and having difficulties. As with alcohol, if a client appears impaired, she may need to make arrangements to get home safely without driving, or she may need medical attention.

Not Completing Homework

Completing between-session homework is a marker of motivation, good rapport with the therapist, effort to practice skills learned in session, treatment retention, and positive treatment outcome. Not completing homework is *not* a reason to terminate therapy. However, homework is an important and unique aspect of CBT and is especially important to help clients practice and consolidate skills in "real life." You should highlight the importance of homework explicitly by reviewing the rationale for it. You also can highlight the importance of homework by reviewing assigned and completed homework carefully and in a clinically meaningful way so that the client feels reinforced for completing her homework. Each group session includes time devoted to the review of homework.

Managing the Group: Common Issues

Group Process

In a group setting, the therapist faces a particular challenge in meeting clinical responsibilities to an individual group member while also addressing issues therapeutically for all members of the group. Therapists should always consider how to harness the power of the group, the lived experience of group members, their ability to empathize and support each other, and, at times, their ability to provide useful suggestions drawn from their common experiences (see Sobell & Sobell, 2011; Yalom, 2005). Group therapy is most successful when the members are encouraged to interact, give feedback, and provide support to one another. You should ask open-ended questions such as, "So, what does the group think about how X handled that high-risk situation?" or "How have others handled a similar situation?" Also, addressing "universality"—group members' feeling that they have problems similar to one another and are not alone in their struggle—is key to building group cohesion and facilitating a healthy group process.

Managing Time

To facilitate group interaction and cover all the skills effectively, therapists provide structure, establish group norms and appropriately intervene, and are mindful to redirect group interaction when needed. Starting with Session 1, orient group members to the agenda for the session and explain that each session has a structured flow. Review the treatment contract in Session 1 and highlight group rules to proactively address time management and group interaction concerns (e.g., arriving on time, turning off cellphones, not interrupting other members or the therapist, not using verbal or physical intimidation). Also inform clients that at times during the session, you may move on to be able to hear from all group members or cover a skill. Group members typically are receptive to this approach and at times have reminded other group members or even the therapist to follow these expectations. The Therapist Guide provides suggested time allotted to each intervention in every session.

Managing Group Members

Group therapy theorists, clinicians, and researchers have described types of group disruption, challenging clients, and ways to manage these (e.g., Sobell & Sobell, 2011; Yalom, 2005). Generally, being aware of different types of potentially challenging behaviors is important. Common challenging behaviors include, for instance, clients who rarely speak in group, consistently arrive late, are interruptive/disruptive, dominate the conversation, give feedback to others but never talk about themselves, are vague and evasive about reporting their substance use, communicate verbally or nonverbally that they are unhappy being in the group, and/or provide confrontational or nonconstructive feedback to others. Having a strategy for handling each type of situation is helpful—such as noticing, validating, and summarizing, and then opening it up to the group or shifting attention from the speaker (see Sobell & Sobell, 2011).

Relationships Among Group Members

The therapist may encourage group members to provide appropriate and alcohol/drug-focused support to one another outside of the group, if deemed clinically advisable. Romantic relationships between women in the group while they are part of the group are generally discouraged, with the rationale that the focus of treatment is better spent on learning skills and obtaining support to achieve and maintain abstinence and overall well-being, as well as developing autonomy and self-efficacy for coping well with challenging situations and feelings.

CHAPTER 5

The Initial Interview: Assessing Alcohol and Drug Use and Problems

Overview of Assessment

This chapter provides an approach to assessment with women who might be good candidates for the women's therapy group described in this Therapist Guide. We provide a description of the initial interview and assessment, detailed suggestions for topics to include in the initial clinical interview, and self-report questionnaires that may be helpful in the assessment. Tailor the assessment to the treatment setting in which the group will be held. Table 5.1 provides a complete list of assessment measures, with recommendations for measures to use in each setting. Finally, we provide some heuristics for clinical decision-making and how to discuss next steps with the client.

As the therapist, you should meet with each potential group member for an assessment session before she joins the group. Prior to the in-person assessment session, clients should be given self-report measures to complete either at home, online, or in the waiting room. You will want to review these self-report questionnaires before meeting with the client. The initial assessment has up to seven major goals, depending on the setting in which the client is seen:

1. To evaluate the client's problems with alcohol and drugs to determine whether and which treatment for alcohol use disorder (AUD) or substance use disorder (SUD) is appropriate, while also determining if the woman is an appropriate candidate to join the women's treatment group described in this guide

2. To determine whether the client has severe medical or psychological problems that require immediate and urgent attention

3. To assess the level of care and services the client needs

Table 5.1. Domains of Assessment, Instruments, and Treatment/Setting-Specific Recommendations (see also Appendix 1)

Assessment Domain	Instrument and Type of Assessment (Interview or Self-Report)	Outpatient Setting	Post-Detoxification Transitional Setting (e.g., Intensive Outpatient Program)	Residential Treatment (e.g., Inpatient Rehabilitation, Sober House, Halfway House)
Clinical intake interview:	*Interviews:*			
a. Presenting problems	a. Clinical interview	a. Necessary	a. Necessary	a. Necessary
b. Current problem substances	b. Clinical interview	b. Necessary	b. Necessary	b. Necessary
c. Overview of alcohol and drug use history	c. Clinical interview	c. Necessary	c. Necessary	c. Necessary
d. Current/recent use	d. Clinical interview	d. Necessary	d. Necessary	d. Necessary
e. Lifetime drug use	e. Lifetime drug use chart	e. Necessary	e. Necessary	e. Necessary
f. DSM-5 AUD/ SUD diagnoses	f. SCID-5-CV (Structured Clinical Interview for DSM-5, Clinician Version)	f. Necessary	f. Necessary	f. Necessary
g. Typical weekly pattern of alcohol and drug use	g. Weekly use grid	g. Necessary	g. Necessary	g. Necessary
h. Daily drug/alcohol use (3 months)	h. Timeline Followback interview	h. Necessary	h. Necessary	h. Necessary
i. Mental health problems/ diagnoses	i. Clinical interview	i. Necessary	i. Necessary	i. Optional
j. Medical problems/ diagnoses	j. Clinical interview	j. Necessary	j. Necessary	j. Optional
k. Other life stressors	k. Clinical interview	k. Necessary	k. Necessary	k. Optional
l. Readiness to change	l. Readiness Rulers	l. Necessary	l. Necessary	l. Necessary
Demographic information	*Self-report*	Necessary	Necessary	Optional

Table 5.1. Continued

Assessment Domain	Instrument and Type of Assessment (Interview or Self-Report)	Outpatient Setting	Post-Detoxification Transitional Setting (e.g., Intensive Outpatient Program)	Residential Treatment (e.g., Inpatient Rehabilitation, Sober House, Halfway House)
Consequences of use	*Self-report:* DrINC (Drinker Inventory of Consequences) and InDUC (Inventory of Drug Use Consequences)	Optional	Optional	Optional
Drinking/drug use goals	*Self-report:* Personal drinking/drug use goals	Necessary	Necessary	Optional
Psychiatric screening	*Self-report:* Beck Depression Inventory *and* Burns Anxiety Inventory, *or* APA DSM-5 screener (American Psychiatric Association Diagnostic and Statistical Manual of Mental Disorders-5 *or* OQ-45.2 (Outcomes Questionnaire-45)	Necessary	Necessary	Necessary
Screening for post-traumatic stress disorder (PTSD)	*Self-report:* PCL-5 (PTSD Checklist for DSM-5)	Necessary	Necessary	Optional
Medications	*Self-report*	Necessary	Necessary	Optional
Hospitalizations	*Self-report*	Necessary	Optional	Optional
Family psychiatric and addiction history	*Self-report*	Optional	Optional	Optional

4. To help with subsequent abstinence planning

5. To collect information that will become the basis for treatment interventions provided in the therapy group, such as assessment feedback and functional analysis

6. To engage and further motivate the client to work toward change in her alcohol and drug use

7. To collect information to help your overall clinical decision-making.

We recommend that you give brief feedback regarding the assessment information to the client at the end of the assessment about whether and what type of treatment is indicated at this time. You will be providing more detailed feedback in Session 1 (Chapter 6) if the woman joins the group. In the cognitive behavioral therapy (CBT) model, continued assessment and a feedback loop throughout treatment are important aspects of the treatment. These are accomplished via daily self-monitoring cards (see Session 1) completed by clients throughout the program that are reviewed each week at the start of the session. Assessment to complete a functional analysis of the client's drinking or drug use occurs as part of the treatment itself and is accomplished in the first two or three sessions.

Assessment Plan

Assessment typically requires approximately 1.5 to 2 hours, depending on the severity of the client's alcohol and drug problems and complications such as comorbid psychopathology and/or social service needs. The assessment includes (see Table 5.1 and below for details):

1. Completion of self-report questionnaires

2. Alcohol/drug testing (breathalyzer, saliva strips, and/or urine drug screen)

3. Unstructured conversation to establish rapport and assess the woman's initial level of motivation

4. Clinical intake interview, including drinking/drug use data, a formal diagnostic interview, and other screening interview questions as needed

5. Therapist review and integration of assessment information

6. Brief feedback and treatment planning with the client.

In this treatment program, assessment is considered to be the start of therapy; it is important to keep in mind that in some settings this may be the first time the client is speaking openly, or speaking at all, about her alcohol and/or drug use. The assessment sessions thus may be difficult and emotional for the client, and it is important for you to establish rapport and to communicate accurate empathy with her perspective, while moving the interview forward and gathering all necessary information.

Clinical Intake Interview

Self-Report Questionnaires

Prior to the clinical intake interview, the client should complete a general demographics form and other self-report questionnaires appropriate to the specific setting (see Table 5.1 for site-specific measures and Appendix I for the self-report measures).

Testing for Presence of Alcohol or Drugs

At the beginning of the clinical intake interview, and at the start of all subsequent sessions, we recommend that the therapist test the client's blood alcohol level (BAL) using a breathalyzer or saliva strip, and do a urine or saliva drug screen for clients who present with drug problems. Clients should be informed of this procedure when scheduling their initial appointment. They should be told that they should come to the appointment alcohol- and drug-free, and that their appointment will be rescheduled should they test positive.

You may introduce the alcohol and drug testing as follows:

My approach is to use an objective measure to check for alcohol (and drugs) in your system. It is important to have a clear head during our meetings together. This means you should not drink alcohol or use any drugs on the day of a scheduled therapy appointment. We will start each session by using this machine/saliva strip to measure your blood alcohol level and to assess for drugs in your body. [If using a breathalyzer: *It is easy to use. I will hold it up to your mouth and you simply take a deep*

breath and blow through the tube for a few seconds until I tell you to stop.
If it seems helpful, you may demonstrate use of the breathalyzer.]

If the client has a positive BAL result or a positive drug screen, ask about her drinking or drug use that day, and for alcohol, explain the relationship between amount of drinking and BAL. If her BAL is above .05, further assess her drinking pattern and consider whether she needs a detoxification program; if this does not seem indicated, reschedule the interview. A positive drug test is more difficult to interpret since many psychoactive drugs stay in the body for several days. You will need to assess the client's clinical status, and if she shows no signs of intoxication or confusion, then you can proceed with the assessment.

The Interview

Spend a few minutes establishing general rapport to help the client feel comfortable through small talk, and then move into the clinical intake interview (see Appendix II). The start of the interview will give the client the opportunity to "tell her story." During this part of the assessment, you should follow the client's lead and listen carefully to judge her motivation for treatment and for change. During the intake interview, you should use therapeutic skills consistent with the spirit of motivational interviewing (MI; Miller & Rollnick, 2013)—for instance, express empathy, maintain a nonjudgmental stance, provide reflections of what the client has said, support "change talk," and use double-sided reflections that acknowledge the client's ambivalence about change but pair her hesitancy about change with reasons for change that she has expressed. However, keep in mind that the intake interview has two primary aims—to enhance/maintain the client's motivation for change and to assess her current functioning and presenting problems to determine the appropriate level of care and appropriateness for the Women's CBT Group for SUD; thus, it is important to stay on task to complete the interview. Use Appendix II to assess and document the problems the client describes (alcohol-related or otherwise). Since you will likely use this form with more than one client, it can be photocopied from the book as needed. Alternatively, assessment forms and client worksheets can be accessed by searching for this book's title on the Oxford Academic platform, at academic.oup.com.

The questions in the intake interview will provide information on the woman's general patterns of drinking and/or drug use as well as her recent and past history. Some of the questions are very detailed. This information is needed for you to calculate the number of standard drinks consumed, as well as approximate BAL for feedback in Session 1 (Chapter 6). It is more difficult to quantify drug use for street drugs because quantities and purities vary considerably, but it is important to assess the pattern of drug use and obtain typical quantities of use in as much detail as much as possible for feedback in Session 1.

Clinical Decision-Making

After completing the initial interviews and structured assessment, you will have a series of decisions to make with the client about treatment planning, depending on the treatment setting and the client's current drinking/drug use status. As a therapist, it is helpful to ask yourself a number of questions:

1. Is the client willing to engage in or continue with treatment at this time?
2. Does the client have any urgent needs that require immediate attention? These might include clear suicidal intent, acute psychosis, an acute and severe medical problem such as chest pain, or living in a situation where she is experiencing severe intimate partner violence.
3. Is the client in need of supervised detoxification before starting in the group?
4. If the group is being offered in an outpatient setting, is the client appropriate for an outpatient group?
5. Does the client have additional psychological problems that would benefit from treatment adjunctive to the therapy group?
6. Does the client have social service needs (e.g., housing, food assistance)?
7. Is the client a good candidate for the group?

Readiness for Change

Virtually all clients presenting for AUD/SUD treatment are ambivalent about changing their alcohol or drug use patterns. The assessment process itself typically helps a client recognize the need for change. The last part of the intake interview includes three *Readiness Rulers* to assess her current motivation for change. If a client responds with a low rating such as 1 or 2 to any of these questions, a follow-up question might be, *"What would make this a 2 or a 3?"* The client's answers to these questions may stimulate further discussion focused on enhancing motivation to change that may be necessary before making a decision about any specific treatment. If a client responds with a high rating (7, for instance), you might ask, *"What made you rate this a 7?"* That question should elicit further change talk and will help consolidate motivation to change her drinking or drug use.

Urgent/Emergency Situations

Few clients presenting to an outpatient setting will have emergency care needs, and clients in aftercare or residential settings typically will not have any emergency care needs, but if the client is acutely suicidal, in severe physical distress (i.e., visible distress that would lead you to tell a friend to go to the emergency room), or acutely psychotic, you should arrange for immediate transport to an emergency room. If the woman is in a living situation with severe intimate partner violence, work with her to develop a safety plan.

Need for Detoxification

During the assessment, you will have obtained information from the Structured Clinical Interview for DSM-5 Disorders, Clinician Version (SCID-5-CV) (First et al., 2016) about withdrawal symptoms. To further assess need for detoxification and to make a level-of-care determination, you should take into account the last time the client had an alcoholic beverage or drug that has associated withdrawal symptoms and ask, *"Are you currently feeling any of these withdrawal symptoms? If so, which ones?"*

Determination of need for detoxification is complex and based on multiple criteria. Some useful guidelines include:

1. Daily drinkers or drug users are more likely to need detoxification than episodic drinkers or users.

2. Morning drinking or drug use or morning withdrawal symptoms suggest a need for detoxification.
3. Persons who drink or use substances on and off throughout the day are more likely to need detoxification than those who drink or use only in the evening.
4. High-volume drinkers who achieve a BAL above .20 to .25 are likely to need detoxification.
5. Persons with a history of withdrawal symptoms who are drinking or using regularly are likely to need detoxification.
6. Persons with a history of withdrawal seizures or major withdrawal syndrome (disorientation, hallucinations) *must* get a medically supervised detoxification.
7. Regular drinkers or drug users who have other medical problems (e.g., history of stroke, high blood pressure, or liver disease) should have a medically supervised detoxification.

If you conclude that the client will need detoxification, this must be addressed at the conclusion of the interview. See Session 1 (Chapter 6) for an overview of abstinence plans, including consideration of types of detoxification plans.

Determining Level of Care

Level-of-care determination depends on several variables based on the severity of recent alcohol/drug problems, medical history, and history of withdrawal symptoms; psychiatric problems; past treatment experiences; support network; insurance considerations; and client preference (see McCrady & Epstein, 2021). In general, the treatment model in this guide is appropriate:

1. As an aftercare program for clients who initially need a medically supervised detoxification
2. For women who do not need or refuse an inpatient detoxification program but meet criteria for alcohol or other substance dependence *or* who are considered to be heavy drinkers because they drink more than 3 standard drinks per occasion or more than 7 per week (note that definitions of heavy drinking for men are different: more than 4 standard drinks per occasion or more than 14 per week) (National Institute on Alcohol Abuse and Alcoholism, 2021a)

3. For clients who do not need inpatient or intensive outpatient treatment
4. For clients who are appropriate for a higher level of care but either cannot or will not seek more intensive services.

In all cases, clients should not have uncontrolled current psychiatric symptoms such as psychosis, mania, or suicidal ideation with intent or plan. Use the results of the assessment to determine the appropriate initial level of care for the client. If the client needs detoxification or an initial course of inpatient treatment, the group would serve as appropriate aftercare. Options for initial abstinence plans (including levels of care) are described in Session 1 (Chapter 6).

Additional Client Needs

In an outpatient setting, the client may have additional needs, including treatment for other psychological problems, interpersonal or relationship issues, social service needs (e.g., housing or food assistance), or medical/health issues. At times, these other issues may be so prominent or pressing that the client would not be able to benefit from the therapy group. More often, however, the therapist will want to develop an integrated care plan to ensure that the woman receives treatment or assistance for these additional issues while participating in the group. For some psychological issues such as depression or anxiety treatment for the alcohol or drug use through the therapy group may resolve these issues; for others, continuing individual treatment or referral to an outside provider would be appropriate.

Appropriateness for Group Therapy

There is a paucity of literature to guide decision-making about the appropriateness of a client for AUD/SUD group therapy, and the literature that exists is contradictory (e.g., Grundmann et al., 2021). Although there is some evidence that women affiliate most successfully in a women-only AUD/SUD therapy group (Valeri et al., 2018), no research provides guidance about who is most likely to affiliate. Contraindications to participation in the group might include difficulty communicating in English, disruptive behavioral disorders, or psychotic features.

Giving Recommendations to the Client

At the end of the assessment, it is important to give the client feedback and to engage her actively in the decision to continue with treatment. If you determine that the client is appropriate for the group and she expresses interest in participating in treatment, you can provide an overview of the therapy group, emphasizing the ways in which you think it could be helpful to her, tailoring your feedback to what you learned during the assessment. You also should ask the client to make an appointment with her physician to get a check-up and bloodwork to assess her current health status. If the client will be joining the group after Session 1 (i.e., at any session between 2 and 12), the therapist should spend an additional 30 minutes with each woman to provide a brief session orientation (described in Chapter 3), to provide the Client Workbook, and to review basic information covered in Session 1 that the client will need to know to proceed with all subsequent sessions.

Need for Detoxification

If you determine that the client needs a supervised detoxification before starting in the group, you should provide feedback about the need for detoxification, tailoring the specific content to the woman's situation. You can then review options, including medication-assisted versus supervised non–medication-assisted detoxification, inpatient versus ambulatory detoxification, or gradual tapering over time.

Recommend inpatient detoxification as the only option if the client has a history of withdrawal seizures or major withdrawal syndrome, or has significant medical problems. Chapter 4 discusses abstinence versus moderate drinking goals for this treatment approach and gives suggestions for how to present the advantages of abstinence.

Summary

Assessment is a pivotal and integral part of CBT for alcohol and drug use problems. This chapter has provided an assessment plan that includes suggested areas to evaluate that are relevant to the treatment of alcohol and drug use problems, as well as specific questions to ask in a clinical interview and recommendations for self-report measures. The assessment will be more or less comprehensive depending on the setting in which the group is offered. Clients who are in residential programs or who would be joining the group as an aftercare treatment will require a less comprehensive assessment than clients entering the group as new clients in an outpatient setting. Guidelines for clinical decision-making for treatment planning and suggestions for providing feedback to the client are included, and more detailed guidance about how to use the assessment data is outlined in Session 1 (Chapter 6). This assessment should allow the therapist to obtain a detailed alcohol and drug history and a clear picture of the woman's current use and negative consequences of that use. The information obtained will allow you to determine the level of care and services needed and to develop an abstinence plan. Clients often find the assessment phase of the treatment to be a valuable and therapeutic way to begin to examine their maladaptive patterns of use.

CHAPTER 6

Session 1: Orientation, Daily Monitoring, and Abstinence Plans

(Corresponds to Chapter 1 in the Client Workbook)
(2 hours)

Notes to the Therapist Before the Session

1. For rolling-admission groups (see Chapter 3), each new member should have an individual assessment (see Chapter 5) with the group facilitator prior to joining the group. At the end of the assessment session, for women joining the group at any session (i.e., Session 2–12) after Session 1, the therapist should spend an additional 30 minutes with each new group member to provide the Client Workbook and to review basic information covered in Session 1 that the client will need to know to proceed with all subsequent sessions. This includes coverage of use of the workbook (see instructions for this in Session 1) and group rules, as well as a brief review of core treatment elements, including self-monitoring, psychoeducation, high-risk situations, triggers, and behavior chains (see Session 2). That way, no matter what session the new member is entering, she will be able to do daily self-monitoring and understand the basics of high-risk situations, triggers, and behavior chains.

2. Each rolling-admission group session with a new member starts with a 5-minute round robin introduction of each group member, and 10 minutes of assessment feedback to the new member(s) (see Session 1 for detailed instructions and feedback sheets). Members in the group at different stages of recovery can provide support to the new client and share their own feedback from their first session. If a new member is lacking relevant information from previous sessions,

she can review sessions in the Client Workbook or you can briefly describe the section, and/or abstinent members can be encouraged to spend time with the new member after session to explain relevant prior material.

3. If this is a client's first session, you must summarize data from the pretreatment assessment to fill in a Feedback Sheet (see Handout 1.10 in Client Workbook) for each client in the group in preparation for her first session.

4. Before the session begins, write the session agenda on a flipchart, whiteboard, or blackboard.

5. If you are doing the Optional Graphing Intervention, see instructions in Chapter 3 of this Therapist Guide.

6. All worksheets and handouts used in this treatment program appear in this Therapist Guide and in the corresponding Client Workbook; worksheets (and selected handouts) can also be accessed by searching for this book's title on the Oxford Academic platform, at academic.oup.com.

Session 1 Outline

All times are approximate and should be adjusted based on clinical need and whether group time needs to be devoted to new or departing members.

1. Pre-session sign-in and substance use check (15 minutes before session begins)

2. Therapist introduction and agenda setting (5 minutes)

3. Introduction of group members (15 minutes)

4. Provide workbook, review treatment requirements and group contract (5 minutes)

5. If there are group members who have already been attending these group sessions, do weekly check-in, review of homework, and (optional) graphing from self-monitoring cards (10 minutes)

6. Treatment rationale, importance of homework and attendance, and psychoeducation on female alcohol use disorder (AUD) and other substance use disorders (SUDs; 10 minutes)

7. Feedback from the intake assessment (20 minutes)

8. Introduction to self-monitoring (15 minutes)

9. Abstinence plans for women still drinking or using drugs and/or other possible problem areas (20 minutes)

10. Farewell to members leaving the group (10 minutes)

11. Anticipating high-risk situations this week (15 minutes)

12. Assign homework (5 minutes)

Materials Needed

1. Flipchart, whiteboard, or blackboard, felt-tip markers or chalk, eraser

2. Breathalyzer and tubes or saliva strips (optional)

3. Saliva drug tests for each group member (optional)

4. Seven self-monitoring cards for each group member (Note to therapist: Keep a stack of these to give group members at each session.)

5. OPTIONAL: Individualized graph for each woman

6. Treatment contract and group rules

7. Completed Feedback Sheet for each client

8. Handouts

   1.1: Treatment Contract

   1.2: Gender Differences in Drinking and Drug Use

   1.3: The Journey Begins

   1.4: The Plan

   1.5: The Importance of Attendance

   1.6: Skills-Based Practice Assignments (aka Homework)

   1.7: Alcohol Information

   1.8a: Percentile Table for Alcohol Use

   1.8b: Percentile Table for Other Drug Use

   1.9: Blood Alcohol Level Estimation Charts

   1.10: Feedback Sheet

   1.11: What Is Self-Monitoring?

   1.12: Self-Monitoring Cards (Instructions and a Completed Example)

   1.13: Self-Monitoring Cards

   1.14: High-Risk Situations: Sample

9. Worksheets

   1.1: Abstinence Plan

   1.2: High-Risk Situations [see Client Workbook Worksheet 1.2]

If any member of the group appears to be high or intoxicated, you may want to assess her blood alcohol level (BAL) with a breathalyzer or saliva strip or use a saliva drug screen. Regardless of formal testing, though, if a group member is visibly high or intoxicated, review the treatment agreement with her and let her know that she will not be allowed to attend this session. Clients who miss a session will not receive a make-up session, but encourage them to read the handouts they missed for that session and complete the homework for the following week. You should assist the client in arranging alternate transportation home, review her abstinence plan, and remind her of her abstinence goal.

Therapist Introduction and Agenda Setting (5 minutes)

Introduce yourself and then provide an overview of Session 1 and set the agenda. To get to know the clients, explain the group therapy process (sharing information with the group and getting feedback from each other in a nonjudgmental manner), discuss the clients' drinking patterns and motivation, and discuss with the clients the rationale for treatment and what the sessions will be like. If the group includes clients who have been in the group and for whom it is not their first session, indicate that we will be reviewing their weekly homework and progress (e.g., daily monitoring cards) as well.

Acknowledge the perceptions and concerns the clients express, particularly with regard to sharing personal drinking or drug use information in a group format. Start setting up the expectation that group members will be doing a lot of the work and that everyone in the group learns by hearing the experiences and advice of others. Encourage group members to direct their comments to the other group members, and not only to you.

Here's how you could introduce the group:

An important part of this treatment is that you will be sharing your experiences with the group. It is important to be open and honest in sharing information, as well as being accepting, nonjudgmental, and non-confrontational when listening to and providing help to each other about your experiences.

The group can be a better therapist than any one individual. I will encourage you to talk to each other, and not just me.

This group format may be more structured than other groups you have been in. The format and content are based on years of research to develop an effective treatment for women struggling with alcohol and/or drug use. We will cover a lot of material in each session. There will also be plenty of time to talk and share your experiences related to the content we are covering, and to support and help each other. More on that later.

EXERCISE 1.1
Introduction of Group Members (15 minutes)

Each group member should be asked to introduce herself and give her name, a bit of information about herself, and what her concerns are about her drinking and/or drug use.

> *Let's go around the room in what we call "round robin style" and have each of you briefly tell us a bit about yourself and also what your concerns are about your drinking and/or drug use. Let's take about 15 minutes now for introductions, so please try to keep your introduction brief (about 2 minutes). I might have to stop you if we're going over time, but we'll have plenty of time to get to know each other as the group progresses.*

Some suggested follow-up questions if clients are reticent:

1. *Tell us a bit about yourself. What is your living situation like (children, extended family, etc.)? How do you spend your time (what kind of work do you do?)*

2. *What concerns do you have about your drinking or drug use?*

3. *What has your drinking/drug use been like over the last couple of weeks?*

Therapist Note

Listen for possible urgent issues that group members might need immediate help with, such as domestic violence, or an acute mood or anxiety disorder. You should address the issue to the degree that appears to be clinically appropriate. Check the guidelines for dealing with urgent issues provided in Chapter 4 *of this guide.*

Be sure to have information from the prior assessment about each group member's frequency and quantity of alcohol consumption and/or drug use in the past 2 weeks to help with abstinence planning at the end of the session.

Provide Workbook, Review Treatment Requirements and Group Contract (5 minutes)

Distribute a workbook to each group member.

This is your own personal workbook to use during each session and between sessions as well. It includes handouts and worksheets for each session. Handouts review the material we cover in session. Worksheets are interactive, and by using them, you will apply the skills learned in session to your own situation. You will start completing the worksheets in session and finish the worksheets at home during the week. The workbook is your own private property—keep it somewhere safe and secure at home, and bring it with you to group each week.

Next, review Handout 1.1: Treatment Contract and have the group members follow along. Stress that there is no rescheduling if a member misses a session, since the groups will be held every week for 12 weeks and follow a specific treatment plan from session to session. If you are holding this as a rolling-admission ("open") group, let group members know that they can continue in the group even after attending 12 sessions. (Also see Chapters 3 and 5 for information on how to handle entry of new members to the group after Session 1.) Expectations for clients include attending all sessions, being on time, providing notification to you at least 24 hours in advance if they cannot attend, not drinking or using drugs for at least 12 hours before the session, and completing homework.

Have the clients read and sign the treatment contract at this time. The clients should be asked to contact you during the week if any problems arise. You should provide clients with your contact information. After going over the treatment contract, ask members if they have any questions. Possible questions to anticipate include:

- **Question:** What if I am sick and unable to attend?

THERAPIST: *Unfortunately, it won't be possible to reschedule group sessions. If you miss a session, you should look at the information in the workbook for that session and try to complete the homework on your own so you can discuss it at the next session. And/or perhaps a group member would be able to review with you what was covered in the missed session.*

■ **Question:** Am I allowed to see or call other group members outside of treatment?

THERAPIST: *We do not discourage outside contact with other group members, but contact is up to you and must of course be mutually acceptable to each person. We do ask that you let the group know if you have spent time with another group member(s) during the week, so that no one gets the feeling that people are keeping secrets from one another. We do discourage forming romantic relationships with other group members while you are both still group members. It's best to focus on your recovery while you're in this treatment.*

■ **Question:** Can we distribute a list of our phone numbers/email addresses?

THERAPIST: *That is entirely up to the group. If someone would like to organize that, I would neither discourage nor encourage that. I just ask that you respect the wishes of those group members who do not feel comfortable distributing their contact information to other members.*

HANDOUT 1.1
Treatment Contract

This treatment will include 12 group sessions over 3 months and I agree to participate for that length of time. If I think about stopping the program at any time, I agree to discuss this decision with the group and therapist *prior* to taking this action.

- I agree to attend *all* sessions. As much as possible, I will make travel, vacation, and other plans *around* group attendance for the next 12 weeks.
- I understand that I must work on being abstinent, clean, and sober during the course of this therapy.
- It is essential for me to come to the session alcohol- and drug-free. I will be asked to leave any session that I come to showing signs that I am intoxicated or high. I will be required to arrange safe transportation home.
- I may be given a breath test for alcohol use before sessions, and possibly a drug test.
- I will be expected to practice the skills discussed in treatment and will complete homework assignments between sessions. I will bring my workbook each week.
- I will respect all group members' confidentiality. That means I will not discuss anything discussed in group outside of the room, except to other group members or the therapist(s) and not in a public place.
- I will be respectful of the therapist and other group members. I will not interrupt other people when they are speaking. I will stop speaking if the group therapist asks me to stop. I will not hold side conversations (cross-talk) with other group members during group. If I am disrespectful to others, I will be asked to leave the room.
- I understand that this must be a safe place for all to talk and discuss personal things. I will be respectful, gentle, supportive, non-confrontational, constructive, and nonjudgmental in my feedback to other group members.
- I will not leave the session for any reason other than emergency. (I will be mindful to use the facilities before the session starts, for instance.)
- I will keep my cellphone turned off during the group session.
- I have the right to say I'd rather just listen for now, if someone directs a question or comment to me that I prefer not to answer.
- I will arrive 15 minutes early for each session to sign in, hand in my daily drinking/drug logs, and possibly have an alcohol and/or a drug test.

I have reviewed the above statements and agree to abide by them.

_____   _____
Client Name   Date

_____   _____
Therapist Name   Date

Check-In, Review of Self-Monitoring and Homework (30 minutes)

Check-in follows a "round robin" format, in which drinking status and homework are emphasized. To introduce the round robin check-in:

We're going to go around the room using what we call a "round robin check-in" to get a brief version of how your week has been, focusing on your alcohol use, drug use, cravings, and triggers; how you coped with triggers and cravings; in hindsight what you might have done differently (with therapist and group input/ideas as well); homework you completed and what was helpful about it. We also will answer or clarify any questions or concerns about the homework material. Each group member will have a few minutes [depending on how many women there are in the group] *to discuss with the group how your coping with alcohol/drug use triggers has been this week.*

Therapist Note

Try to pay particular attention to women's specific themes (e.g., right to self-care, empowerment) and link experiences to the specific themes: "One theme I've heard that's common among several of you is . . ."

Go around the room and ask each group member how her week was (focusing on alcohol and/or drug use); listen while looking over her self-monitoring cards; and link what she is saying to her daily cards for alcohol/drug cravings, triggers, and use. Use information from this for specific topics in the rest of the session. Check in with each group member and discuss the progress of her abstinence plan. Update the plan if necessary. Also remember to ask each client at the end of her round robin time about what homework she was able to complete.

You should reinforce self-recording behavior, check for questions or problems, and help group members develop solutions for difficulties related to self-recording procedures. Ask members if they have any questions. Possible questions to anticipate include:

- **Question:** I thought about drinking the whole morning. Is that one urge or more than one?

THERAPIST: *You had the urge continually?*

CLIENT: Not every minute.

THERAPIST: *Well, each time you have a thought or an image about having a specific type of drink or a drink in a particular situation, that counts as a separate urge. Can you share some specific situations you thought about?*

▪ **Question:** Why are my urges so much stronger than everyone else's? Why am I the only one still drinking?

THERAPIST: *It's natural that you would want to compare your drinking/drug use and urges to those of the other group members. Although this can be an important motivator, it also is important to remember that everyone has her own unique path to abstinence. You're working on it, so be patient with yourself, and think of the changes you've already made! What does the group think about what _____ said?*

Therapist Note
After reviewing the daily monitoring cards, for outpatient settings you may wish to include the optional Graphing Intervention here.

Optional Graphing Intervention for Outpatient Treatment Settings

See the detailed instructions in Chapter 3 of this guide for how to use the graphs located in Session 2 of the Therapist Guide and in the Client Workbook (Handout 2.1: Graph: Alcohol/Drug Use and Urges Sample and Worksheet 2.1: Graph: Alcohol/Drug Use and Urges). This intervention will allow each woman to track her progress by entering weekly data summarized from her daily monitoring cards: 1. Number of drinks; 2. Number of drugs used; 3. Number of urges/cravings; and 4. Average strength of urges/cravings.

Other Homework Review

Review all other homework clients did during the prior week. Reinforce clients for completing their homework and discuss barriers experienced in completing it. Ask questions, such as *"What did you learn from the homework?"* or *"How can you use the homework to help you in the future?"*

Remember that, as part of homework review, each week you need to review group members' recording of high-risk situations and how these were handled: *"Who wants to share how you handled one of your high-risk situations this week without drinking/using drugs?"* Elicit high-risk examples from two or three group members and get feedback from other members. Remember to have group members direct their comments to the other group members, and not just to you. Point out common types of high-risk situations among the group members and encourage women facing similar situations to share how they coped or ideas for coping. Selectively model and repeat empowering and motivational positive affirmations that group members give to one another: for instance, *"We know this is hard, you're doing great." "Next time you'll be able to use a different strategy, hang in there."*

Also, ask about progress with doctor's appointments and blood tests. Due to time constraints, group members should discuss any concerns about their blood tests or feedback with you after the group. Ask each client to bring in a copy of her lab results and give it to you. You can give feedback to the client during review of homework either that week or the week after.

> **Therapist Note**
>
> *You should manage participation so that there is enough time to go around the room in a round robin fashion and give each group member a chance to speak. Keep in mind that 10 to 30 minutes total is allotted for check-in, depending on how many women are in the group. If homework is not done, you should ask what made it difficult for the client to complete the homework. The importance of completing homework should be discussed, and a firm commitment for the future should be stressed in a nonjudgmental way.*

Share the following with the group:

The time in the treatment group is only part of the process. The real change occurs when you practice changing your lives in the real world. The group will help you get ideas, stay motivated, keep you on track, and develop an understanding of the problem. But actually changing behavior takes place in your everyday life—at home, at work, with family, friends, and so on.

Therapist Note

The following are some tips for managing members' participation to maintain the temporal structure of the session. For habitually quiet members or those who appear upset or distressed, you should acknowledge them with empathic nonverbal behavior, but do not call on them to elicit participation right away, except during their turn in the round robin. Look for opportunities to invite limited participation of habitually quiet members to help them become comfortable sharing. Frequently ask the group for their feedback on particular group members' contributions to set up the expectation that group members will be doing a lot of the work in the room. Everyone in the group learns by hearing the experiences and advice of others. Model and facilitate a tone of supportive, constructive, and compassionate feedback in the group. Don't be confrontational, but also don't condone or reassure a woman about her drinking/drug use or lack of work outside the group sessions. For instance, don't say "It's okay. You had a really hard week; of course you drank a bit." Say instead "You certainly had a hard week! In hindsight, what could you have done differently in response to trigger xxx?"

Group members who are having substantial difficulty with their abstinence plan or who appear to be at risk for an emergency should be asked discreetly to remain after group for an individual check-in with you.

Treatment Rationale, Importance of Homework and Attendance, and Psychoeducation on Female Alcohol Use Disorder and Other Substance Use Disorders (10 minutes)

Refer clients to Handouts 1.2: Gender Differences in Drinking and Drug Use, 1.3: The Journey Begins, and 1.4: The Plan.

Why a Female-Specific Alcohol/Drug Treatment Program?

Try to generate some discussion about this information with the group and make the psychoeducational material meaningful by stimulating an interactive exchange.

Here is a way to introduce this discussion:

This treatment is designed specifically for women. There are very few alcohol or drug treatment programs in this country just for women, but we now know there are many differences between men's and women's problem drinking and drug use. Handout 1.2 summarizes some of the unique aspects of women's drinking and drug use, so you can follow along while we discuss.

Ask the group for reactions, opinions, or personal experience with any of these topics.

HANDOUT 1.2
Gender Differences in Drinking and Drug Use

There is a growing body of research showing that female problem drinking and drug use are different on many levels from male problem drinking and drug use. Women in general are at greater risk than men to suffer from several negative consequences of alcohol and drugs.

- Women have less body water and less muscle mass than men, so the concentration of alcohol in their bodies is higher than in men of a similar weight, after drinking the same amounts of alcohol.
- Women experience a "telescoping effect" of alcohol—that is, women's problem drinking generally starts later in life than men's, but women develop problems more quickly than men.
- Women are more vulnerable than men to liver, heart, and brain damage from alcohol or drug use.
- Women are at increased risk for violent victimization when drinking, as well as alcohol-related traffic fatalities.
- Women have a seven-fold increased risk for death from alcohol-related causes, compared to a four-fold increased risk for men.
- Women in general, and particularly women with drinking problems, are at greater risk than men to develop mental health problems, such as depression, anxiety, and eating disorders.
- Women typically are more concerned than men with relationships, self-esteem, and caretaking.
- Women with alcohol use disorder tend to be in relationships with men who drink or have a drinking problem (one-third to one-half of these male partners have an alcohol use disorder).
- Women problem drinkers have more marital disruption than male problem drinkers.
- Women differ from men in terms of triggers to drink, as well as where they drink, their emotions, and their relationships with others. Women are more likely to drink alone and in response to emotional cues and interpersonal cues.
- Following treatment, women have relapse triggers that are different than men.
- Women may become addicted to drugs more quickly than men, even when using smaller amounts.

- Women often have more drug cravings than men.
- Women may be more sensitive to the effects of some drugs than men because of their hormones; their brains, hearts, and blood vessels may be affected differently.
- Women are more vulnerable to drug overdoses than are men.
- Women who experience violence from their partners are at risk for developing drug problems.
- Women may develop drug problems after a divorce, loss of custody of their child, or the death of their partner.
- Women with drug problems also are at risk to develop problems such as anxiety, depression, or panic attacks.
- Drug and alcohol use during pregnancy can harm the developing fetus; babies of mothers who were using opioids during pregnancy may go into withdrawal when they are born.
- Women drug users may be more vulnerable to relapse after treatment.

Introduce the main topics/goals for the treatment program. Walk the group members through Handouts 1.3: The Journey Begins and 1.4: The Plan while they follow along in their workbooks.

HANDOUT 1.3
The Journey Begins

- Together we are starting a journey.
- **The most successful and ambitious journeys all start with a roadmap (a plan) and a destination (a goal).**
- **The roadmap** is this therapy. We will show you ways of quitting drinking and/or drug use and improving your life.
- We will work on identifying **high-risk** situations—those that *may* lead to drinking or drug use. Some of these situations will involve places, people, and things that you come across. Some of these situations will involve thoughts and emotions that are connected to your use. Some of these situations may come from your relationships.
- We will develop a **plan** and **skills** to get through these tough situations.
- This journey will require **dedication**. In each session, we will provide a new skill or technique for dealing with high-risk situations.
- **The road will get bumpy at times.** Sometimes things may be so rough that you will wonder if you've made a wrong turn. Many people who decide to quit drinking or using drugs have a rough time in the beginning. We will look at these rough times as chances to learn more about the kinds of situations that are risky and what it takes to get through them.
- When learning to ride a bicycle, most people will fall a few times. Almost everyone gets back on the bicycle and eventually succeeds in learning to ride. **You may go down the wrong path during our journey. If you do, recognizing this will be important so you can get back on the right road.**
- **One very important part of this therapy is your commitment to working with your therapist and the group.** Each week your therapist will ask you to do things during the week. It is very important that you work hard at home.
- **Many women have succeeded** with this program. The things you'll learn have helped many people stop using alcohol and drugs and build better lives and relationships.

- Study your drinking and drug use habits. Figure out what leads to drinking or drug use and what keeps it going.
- Change habits and things around you that lead to or encourage drinking or drug use.
- Learn positive alternatives to drinking alcohol or using drugs.
- Learn coping skills to enhance and protect your mental health, correct unwanted behaviors, be free of shame, and accept self-compassion and pride.
- Learn skills to enhance and maintain wellness.

Goals of this program are to help you to:

- Become or stay abstinent.
- Anticipate and cope with situations that are high risk for drinking/drug use.
- Learn about the unique challenges that women with drinking/drug problems face.
- Develop a balanced lifestyle that allows time for pleasures and responsibilities.
- Treat yourself and talk to yourself with more compassion.
- Feel like you are in control of your own life.
- Give yourself as much care and caring as you give others.
- Be less emotionally reactive to those around you.
- Cope with feelings of depression, anxiety, anger, and strong negative emotion.
- Feel more connected to others in your life.
- Develop or maintain wellness behaviors and habits.
- Avoid as well as cope with relapses.
- Maintain the new things that you have learned during the treatment.

Ask clients how they feel about the above issues; respond to issues such as minimization of problems, misconceptions about etiology, and lack of taking responsibility for behavior or behavior change, in a nonjudgmental way: *"If you have questions or are having a hard time, please let me know—that's what I'm here for."*

Share the following with the group members, while directing them to Handouts 1.5: The Importance of Attendance and 1.6: Skills-Based Practice Assignments (aka Homework):

*For this therapy to be most helpful, you need to make a very important commitment to be an **active participant** in this process. That means coming to **all** therapy sessions and completing **all** homework assignments.*

HANDOUT 1.5
The Importance of Attendance

- Clients who attend more sessions do better by the end of treatment and over the long term.
- Because this treatment is designed to increase your skill level at handling life without alcohol or drugs, each session builds on previous sessions.
- Regular weekly attendance helps maintain a consistent focus and goal throughout the treatment and maximizes the benefits.
- Attending these sessions is a way of taking care of yourself; make your well-being a priority in life. Your well-being will spread out to enhance that of your children, family, and friends.
- It's a group effort, so your attendance benefits others in the group—and vice versa.

Some strategies for helping you attend every session:

- Arrange at work in advance to protect time to attend the sessions for the next 12 weeks.
- Set aside a 3- to 4-hour block of time for treatment each week: 1.5 hours for group and 30 minutes for early arrival and check-in, which leaves you up to an hour each way for travel to and from the group sessions.
- If needed, arrange carpools with other group members to come to the group together.
- Have back-up transportation plans for situations that arise in which you will not have access to a car.
- Tell your family in advance that you will be busy during this time for the next 12 weeks. Arrange childcare in advance as necessary.
- Remind yourself that coming to therapy every week is no different than following the directions on prescription medication from your doctor—it is important to take it on a consistent basis and not miss a dose!
- Share with the group members if you are having concerns about how to make attendance a priority; we're here to help.
- Be assertive in protecting your right to take care of yourself!

HANDOUT 1.6
Skills-Based Practice Assignments (aka Homework)

Why is practice so important?

◆ Changing your behavior is hard, can be scary, and is unsettling, but if you can manage it, your life is going to be better.

◆ Change doesn't just happen; you have to make it happen via homework.

◆ Part of our focus is to help you take better care of yourself. Between-session assignments are a good way to carve out time for yourself and focus on YOUR OWN NEEDS— something you may have been neglecting for a while now.

◆ There are 168 hours in a week. We have the opportunity to see you for about 2 of those hours; this leaves the rest of the week for you to learn to be your own therapist. Practicing skills outside of session with assignments is the best way to do this.

◆ Practicing in your day-to-day life is a great way to learn "in the moment" how to cope with triggers and cravings in order to stay sober.

◆ It is important to talk about your progress and learn new skills in the group, and also to practice them at home.

◆ The goal is to give you a "toolkit" of new coping skills.

Here are some strategies for helping you to make homework a priority:

◆ *Set aside* 30 or 60 minutes before bedtime or in the morning while you are having your coffee or tea to do your homework.

◆ *Remind yourself* that homework is a way to take care of yourself.

◆ *Consider your homework* "me" time, when you are doing something good and healthy for yourself.

◆ *Set up a consistent place* to do your homework.

◆ *Carry your self-monitoring cards* (refer to Handouts 1.11 to 1.13 later in this session) in your purse so that you can use them to record "in the moment."

◆ *Tell your friends and/or family* that you will be busy at a certain time every day for the next few months, and use that time to do your homework for the week.

For Exercise 1.2, use a round robin to go over Handout 1.10: Feedback Sheet for each client; have clients follow along with the sheets you give them. Briefly review how to calculate standard drinks using Handout 1.7: Alcohol Information, and how to calculate blood alcohol level (BAL) and percentile, using Handouts 1.8a: Percentile Table for Alcohol Use and 1.8b: Past-Year Use of Other Drugs, so that they can understand the feedback. Talk to the group generally while they follow along with their own individual feedback sheets.

Therapist Note

You will need to complete a Feedback Sheet (Handout 1.10) for each group member. This form can be photocopied from the Therapist Guide or the client workbook, or it can be accessed by searching for this book's title on the Oxford Academic platform, at academic.oup.com.

EXERCISE 1.2
Feedback

Paraphrase the following to everyone before the round robin feedback starts:

Based on the information from the assessment session, I summarized your drug use in terms of what kinds of drugs you were using, and how often. I also calculated the number of "standard drinks" you consumed in a typical week, during the 3 months before you started treatment. A standard drink is a unit of measurement for ethanol, the active ingredient in alcohol. Because the ratio of ethanol to non-ethanol liquid in an alcohol beverage is different for different alcoholic beverages, converting to standard drinks allows us to compare units of alcohol across types of drinks and allows us to calculate blood alcohol level. For instance, 5 ounces of wine has approximately 1 unit of ethanol—that is, 1 standard drink—while only 1.5 ounces of vodka is also 1 unit of ethanol (1 standard drink). The higher the "proof" (percentage of ethanol) of the beverage, the less you need to make a standard drink. Vodka typically is 80 proof (40% alcohol), while wine is typically about 13% to 15% alcohol. Regular domestic beer is typically about 5% alcohol, while IPAs are often about 9% alcohol. Light beer has a lower percentage of alcohol, about 4%.

I would like to ask you to share the average number of standard drinks per week you had been consuming, as well as your average number of standard drinks per drinking day. Your feedback sheet for alcohol tells you where this places your drinking in terms of women in America. For example, if you are in the 95th percentile, you have been drinking more than approximately 95% of women in America, and more than 89% percent of adults in America. If you have been using drugs, you can see what percentage of women and adults in the United States use different kinds of drugs. [Refer to Handouts 1.7, 1.8a, and 1.8b here.]

For our purposes, we define "drug" as any illicit drug such as cocaine, heroin, marijuana or other cannabis product, or any addictive medication that is abused (that is, not used as prescribed) such as painkillers or benzodiazepines. We consider use of marijuana or other cannabis products to be illicit drug use because it is illegal federally and in many states; also, all cannabis products are addictive substances that can yield a substance use disorder with associated negative consequences.

I also estimated your peak and typical blood alcohol level (BAL) in the last 3 months. Your BAL (also known as blood alcohol content, or BAC) is based on how many standard drinks you consume, the length of time over which you drink that many standard drinks (we metabolize, that is eliminate, approximately 1 standard drink per hour, so you need to subtract .015 from estimated BAL for every hour you drink), whether you are a male or female, and how much you weigh. So, for instance, if you weigh 140 pounds and drink 10 standard drinks over 2 hours, your BAL would be 0.29%. We use these tables to estimate your BAL for the amount of alcohol you typically drink on a drinking occasion, and your highest BAL for the past 3 months. The BAL is a measure of how intoxicated you typically become. There is a list in your workbook outlining the impairment people suffer based on different BALs. In most states, legal intoxication is considered a BAL of .08% or higher. [Refer to Handout 1.7 and Handout 1.9: Blood Alcohol Level Estimation Charts.]

The point of this exercise is to think about alcohol in a new way—to think about alcohol (or ethanol, which is the active ingredient in alcohol) as a chemical, actually a toxin (poison) that accumulates in our system while we drink and affects our brain. If we consume more alcohol than we can metabolize, as drinking goes on, we get more and more intoxicated. If we drink enough alcohol to outpace metabolism, alcohol poisoning can occur because of a high blood alcohol level. Alcohol poisoning can be fatal.

Have the women go around the room round robin style and share the information that is on their feedback sheet for drinks per week and drinks per drinking day, their typical BAL, and consequences. Solicit group members' reactions to their feedback on alcohol and drug use. You should listen attentively, convey understanding verbally and nonverbally, and indicate that clients with similar drinking and drug problems have successfully utilized this treatment, to help establish positive expectancies.

I know it's hard to take a look at your drinking and drug use in the harsh light of day, and you might feel out of control of some areas of your life now. But you're more in control than you know—because you got yourself here (to treatment). You knew to do that for yourself. Treatment will help you feel more in charge of yourself and your life, which will go a long way to help you feel better about yourself. The next few weeks may be difficult at times, as you stop drinking or using drugs, but it will be worth it. Making time to be here and to work on skills during the week is a way to take care of yourself.

■ **Question:** But how can I find time?

THERAPIST: *If your kids are due for an annual check-up, you make time to take them, right? If your partner or mother needed a blood test, you would be willing to make time and take them. So treat yourself with the same care. Nurture yourself—you deserve it. Make time for yourself to take care of your health needs.*

Therapist Note

*At the individual intake (see Chapter 5), you will have suggested to each client that she should make an appointment to see her physician for a check-up and to get a blood test to check on liver function, since alcohol and other drugs are toxins and can affect the liver and other vital organs. Remind the women about this suggestion and ask them **to bring lab results in to show you.***

Standard Drinks

Beer:

Ounces	Light	Regular	European	Ice	IPAs, Craft
12	0.75	1.00	1.25	1.50	1.50-1.75
16	1.00	1.33	1.66	2.00	2.00-2.33

Spiked Selzer:

One 12-ounce can = 1 standard drink (if alcohol content is about 5%)

Wine:

5 ounces = 1 standard drink; one 750-ml bottle of wine = 5 standard drinks

Hard Liquor:

1.5 ounces of 80-proof liquor = 1 standard drink

Equivalent Number of Standard Drinks

Amount	Street Name	Ounces	80 proof	100 proof	190 proof
	"Shot"	1.5	1	1.25	2.38
200 ml	"Half pint"	6.8	4.5	5.67	10.77
375 ml	"Pint"	12.75	8.5	10.63	20.19
750 m	"Fifth"	25.5	17	21.25	40.38
1.75 L	"Half gallon"	59.5	40	49.58	94.21

Blood Alcohol Level (BAL)

BAL depends on the amount and type of alcohol consumed, over how long a time period it was consumed, whether the person has been eating, and how much person weighs. Effects of BAL on drinker depends in part on physiological tolerance to ethanol.

Common Effects of Different Levels of Blood Alcohol Level for Drinkers

(Adapted from: https://www.niaaa.nih.gov/publications/brochures-and-fact-sheets/understanding-dangers-of-alcohol-overdose, 2021)

.02—.05%: Mild impairment in speech, memory, judgement, coordination, balance. Driving may be unsafe.

.06—.15%: Increased impairment in memory, judgment, speech, balance, coordination, perception, reaction time. Vomiting (signs of alcohol overdose) and blackouts (gaps in memory) may occur. Legally intoxicated above .08 in most states. Significant impairments in all driving skills.

.16—.30%: Severe impairment in all of above. Decision-making and judgment dangerously impaired. Vomiting, blackouts, and/or loss of consciousness likely to occur.

.31—.45%: Danger of life-threatening overdose. Loss of consciousness, high risk of fatal dose.

ALCOHOL CONSUMPTION NORMS FOR U.S. ADULTS

DRINKS PER WEEK	Men*	Women*	Total*
0 (Abstainers)	25%	31%	28%
1	50%	65%	58%
2	61%	74%	67%
3	65%	78%	72%
4	69%	81%	75%
5	72%	84%	78%
6	75%	85%	80%
7	77%	87%	82%
8	80%	88%	84%
9	82%	89%	86%
10	83%	90%	87%
11	85%	91%	88%
12	86%	92%	89%
13	87%	92%	89%
14	88%	93%	90%
15	88%	94%	91%
16-17	89%	94%	92%
18-19	91%	95%	93%
20-21	92%	96%	94%
22-23	92%	97%	94%
24-26	92%	97%	95%
27-30	94%	97%	96%
31-36	95%	98%	96%
37-42	96%	98%	97%
43-49	97%	99%	98%
50-59	97%	99%	98%
60-69	98%	99%	99%
70+	99%	100%	99%

* Results rounded to the nearest percentile.

Source: 2020 National Alcohol Survey of 9,668 individuals. Alcohol Research Group, 6001Shellmound Street, Suite 450, Emeryville, California 94608. www.arg.org

Courtesy of Drs. Thomas K. Greenfield tgreenfield@arg.org and Priscilla Martinez pmartinez@arg.org, National Alcohol Survey, NIAAA-supported Alcohol Research Center Grant (P50AA005595; PI William C. Kerr, PhD); with thanks to Biostatistician Yu Ye yye@arg.org.

HANDOUT 1.8b
Percentile Table for Other Drug Use

This table shows the percentage of men and women in the United States who have used each drug listed at least once in the prior year.

Drug	Men	Women	Total
Any illicit drug	22.7%	16.2%	19.3%
Any illicit drug except marijuana	10.7%	7.6%	9.1%
Marijuana	18.4%	12.4%	15.3%
Opioids (illicit)	5.0%	3.7%	4.3%
Pain relievers (misuse)	4.8%	3.6%	4.2%
Tranquilizers or sedatives	2.6%	2.5%	2.5%
Cocaine	3.3%	1.5%	2.4%
Stimulants	2.7%	1.7%	2.2%
Hallucinogens	2.5%	1.3%	1.9%
Benzodiazepines	1.6%	1.6%	1.6%
Methamphetamines	0.9%	0.4%	0.6%
Inhalants	0.7%	0.3%	0.5%

From: https://www.samhsa.gov/data/sites/default/files/cbhsq-reports/NSDUHDetailedTabs2018R2/NSDUHDet TabsSect1pe2018.htm (accessed 10-19-20)

Blood Alcohol Level Estimation Charts

Men: Approximate Blood Alcohol Percentage

Drinks	Body Weight in Pounds							
	100	120	140	160	180	200	220	240
0	.00	.00	.00	.00	.00	.00	.00	.00
1	.04	.03	.03	.02	.02	.02	.02	.02
2	.08	.06	.05	.05	.04	.04	.03	.03
3	.11	.09	.08	.07	.06	.06	.05	.05
4	.15	.12	.11	.09	.08	.08	.07	.06
5	.19	.16	.13	.12	.11	.09	.09	.08
6	.23	.19	.16	.14	.13	.11	.10	.09
7	.26	.22	.19	.16	.15	.13	.12	.11
8	.30	.25	.21	.19	.17	.15	.14	.13
9	.34	.28	.24	.21	.19	.7	.15	.14
10	.38	.31	.27	.23	.21	.19	.17	.16

Women: Approximate Blood Alcohol Percentage

Drinks	Body Weight in Pounds								
	90	100	120	140	160	180	200	220	240
0	.00	.00	.00	.00	.00	.00	.00	.00	.00
1	.05	.05	.05	.03	.03	.03	.02	.02	.02
2	.10	.09	.08	.07	.06	.05	.05	.04	.04
3	.15	.14	.11	.10	.09	.08	.07	.06	.06
4	.20	.18	.15	.13	.11	.10	.09	.08	.08
5	.25	.23	.19	.16	.14	.13	.11	.10	.09
6	.30	.27	.23	.19	.17	.15	.14	.12	.11
7	.35	.32	.27	.23	.20	.18	.16	.14	.13
8	.40	.36	.30	.26	.23	.20	.18	.17	.15
9	.45	.41	.34	.29	.26	.23	.20	.19	.17
10	.51	.45	.38	.32	.28	.25	.23	.21	.19

One drink is a 1.5-oz shot of hard liquor, 12 oz of domestic beer, or 5 oz of table wine.

Subtract .015 for each hour that you take to consume the drinks. For example, if you are a 140-pound woman and have 3 drinks in 2 hours, estimated BAL would be .07: $(.10 - (2 \times .015) = .07.)$

Blood alcohol level (BAL) charts do not take into account variables such as, water to body mass ratio, ethanol metabolism, tolerance level, or speed of consumption. *Thus, these charts provide only rough estimates.*

Adapted from BAC Charts produced by the National Clearinghouse for Alcohol and Drug Information

Note: You also can calculate your BAL by going to https://casaa.unm.edu/BACcalc.html and entering your sex, weight, type of drink, number of drinks, and number of hours over which you drank.

HANDOUT 1.10
Feedback Sheet

1. Your recent (last 3 months to a year) drug or nicotine use pattern has been to use:

   a. _____ (drug) on _____ days per week, _____ times per day, from _____ to _____.
      Method of administration and potency (level THC, amount, dose): _____.

   b. _____ (drug) on _____ days per week, _____ times per day, from _____ to _____.
      Method of administration and potency (level THC, amount, dose): _____.

   c. _____ (drug) on _____ days per week, _____ times per day, from _____ to _____.
      Method of administration and potency (level THC, amount, dose): _____.

2. In addition to the drugs you used recently, over your lifetime you also have used these other drugs:

   _____

   _____

3. Over the last 3 to 6 months, the number of "standard drinks" you typically drank was:

   Total number of standard drinks per typical *week* _____

   Average number of standard drinks per *drinking day* _____

4. When we look at everyone who drinks in the United States, you have been drinking more than approximately _____ % of the population of women in the country.

5. I also estimated your highest and average blood alcohol level (BAL) in the past 3 months. Your BAL is based on how many standard drinks you consume, the length of time over which you drink that much, whether you are a man or a woman, and how much you weigh.

   Your estimated *peak BAL* in the past 3 months was _____

   Your estimated *typical BAL for drinking days* in an average week was _____

6. You also have some risk factors for having a drug or alcohol problem (examples: family history, other psychological problems, financial problems, legal problems):

   _____

   _____

   _____

7. These are some negative consequences you have experienced from your alcohol or drug use:

   _____

   _____

   _____

Introduction to Self-Monitoring (15 minutes)

Ask members to read Handouts 1.11: What Is Self-Monitoring? and 1.12: Self-Monitoring Cards (Instructions and a Completed Example) while you review the topic.

Rationale:

Self-monitoring is when you track (on paper or an app) the behavior that you want to change. Monitoring your drinking or drug use and urges helps you practice being aware of triggers and mindful of behavior chains, including your response to triggers (i.e., your substance use behavior). The first step in changing your behavior is being aware of it. Also, we know that tracking a behavior is the single best way to change it.

Monitoring helps us identify patterns in your drinking and drug use and how it interfaces with your daily life. With the monitoring cards, we will be able to figure out different chains of behaviors that lead to drinking or drug use.

When people self-monitor, they are often surprised by how much alcohol or drugs they are using. People are also able to see that their drinking or drug use falls into patterns that happen over and over. The self-monitoring also gives us an idea of how often you are getting urges (also called cravings, or desires to drink or use drugs) and what leads to these urges. It also helps you identify your urges/cravings in real time in your daily lives and be more mindful of them. This information will help us make a plan to manage urges to drink or use drugs. Some urges will be tougher to resist than others. You will learn more about which ones are easier to resist than others.

The monitoring will help us see your progress as we go through this program.

On the cards we provide, you should write down your urges (cravings) to drink or use, any drinks or drugs you may have had, and your mood.

You will need to do this every day, throughout the day. I will help you figure out a way to remember to record this every day. One suggestion is to keep the cards I give you in a place with other things that you always have with you. When you have a drink or drug or have an urge, write it down as soon as possible. Don't rely on your memory later.

> **Therapist Note**
>
> *You will provide multiple copies of the self-monitoring cards described in Handout 1.12 to each group member. A blank copy of this card is shown in Handout 1.13: Self-Monitoring Cards; it can be photocopied from the Therapist Guide or the Client Workbook, or it can be accessed by searching for this book's title on the Oxford Academic platform, at academic.oup.com.*

Give the self-monitoring cards to the clients. Ask them to keep a daily record of the following:

- Drinking and drug use
- Cravings (urges) or thoughts about drinking or using drugs (both quantity and strength)
- How many cigarettes they smoked (if applicable)
- An overall mood rating
- How much money they spent on alcohol and drugs that day
- Whether they worked on changing any well-being behavior they are focused on.

Self-monitoring responses should be taught using the flipchart, whiteboard, or blackboard and also through role-playing with a volunteer in order to ensure that the procedures are clearly understood.

Tell clients to carry their cards with them at all times, one per day. If they drink or use a drug, they should record before each drink (i.e., record each drink or drug separately). The clients should include details about what type of drink or drug (e.g., "Bud Light" or "Bud Ice," or "edible"), how much (ounces), and the situation in which the drinking or drug use occurred. Also, they should record each thought or urge immediately and its intensity on a 1-to-7 scale (7 = most intense). Let clients know that urges (cravings) may occur for months after stopping drinking or using drugs, so they shouldn't be surprised.

Briefly review the handouts on self-monitoring with the clients. Then, have the women recall their last drinking or drug use episode and record it on a sample card as practice.

HANDOUT 1.11
What Is Self-Monitoring?

An important part of treatment is to become very aware of your triggers to drink/use, your cravings, and your actual drinking/use so that you can change those behaviors. The best way to track your drinking/drug use is in real time, as the cravings and use happen.

- Self-monitoring is when you track (on paper or an app) the behavior that you want to change. Monitoring your drinking or drug use and urges helps you practice being aware of triggers and mindful of behavior chains, including your response to triggers (i.e., your substance use behavior). The first step in changing your behavior is being aware of it. Also, we know that tracking a behavior is the single best way to change it.
- Monitoring helps us identify patterns in your drinking and drug use and how it interfaces with your daily life. With the monitoring records, we will be able to figure out different chains of behaviors that lead to drinking or drug use.
- With self-monitoring, many women with drinking or drug problems are surprised with how much they are drinking or using and that their drinking or drug use falls into patterns that happen over and over. It also helps us to realize how often you are getting urges or desires to drink or use and what leads to these urges. We will learn how you are able to handle some of these urges already. Some urges will be tougher than others. We will learn more about which ones are easier than others.
- We will also look at how your mood is each day. You should see a general improvement in your mood as this program continues, especially after you stop drinking and are over withdrawal.
- The monitoring will help us see your progress as we go through this program.
- On the cards we provide, you should write down your urges/cravings to drink or use drugs, any drinks or drugs you may have had, and your mood.
- You should do this every day. One suggestion to remember is to keep the cards in a place with other things that you always have with you. When you have a drink or drug or have an urge, write it down as soon as possible.
- You also might want to use an app to keep track of your drinking. We have used the AlcoDroid tracker https://play.google.com/store/apps/details?id=org.M.alcodroid&hl=en) or DrinkControl (https://drinkcontrolapp.com/), but there are many other useful apps available—the important thing is to find one that works for you.

This information that you are collecting is very helpful.

On Handout 1.12, there is an example of a completed self-monitoring card, along with instructions for how to fill out this card. Since completing these cards is so important, we want you to understand how it should be done. If you have questions, talk to your therapist or ask other group members. Then, Handout 1.13 contains a blank self-monitoring card for you to fill out. Your therapist will provide multiple copies of this card for you.

Self-Monitoring Cards (Instructions and a Completed Example)

The self-monitoring cards are an easy way to keep track of what is happening with your urges and drinking or drug use from day to day. There will be a card for every day. Under each section, we ask you to fill in the following information. Write down your urges (cravings) and any actual drinks or drug use. Also rate your mood, write down how many cigarettes you smoked (if any), answer yes/no if you have a wellness behavior goal (such as exercising, eating healthy, doing a pleasant activity you enjoy) in addition to changing your drinking or drug use, and write how much money you spent on alcohol or drugs (if any).

Note: "Urge" means craving to drink/use.

Daily Drink or Drug Use Monitoring				Name__ Sally __ Date__ 7/12/20 __			
Urges/Cravings			**Drinking or Drug use**				
Time	How Strong? (1-7)	Trigger	Time	Drink or Drug	Amount (Drinks in ounces)	% Alcohol	Trigger
8 AM	4	Kids in bad mood all morning					
4 PM	5	Mom called – demanding & tearful					
5:30 PM	7	John irritated when got home	6 PM	Wine	1 bottle	12%	Fight with John

How many cigarettes did you smoke today? __0__

Mood: 1 2 (3) 4 5 6 7
Excellent   Extremely bad/negative

Did you work on a well-being behavior today?   Yes (No) | How much money did you spend on alcohol or drugs today? $15

Date: Make sure to write in the **date** that you are completing the card. You should fill in a card for every day of the week. We will use this information to look at patterns that happen across the week.

Urges/Cravings: Under **Urges/Cravings**, we would like you to write down at what time the urge happened and how intense it was. For intensity, put down a number between 1 and 7 to describe how strong the urge was. Number 1 would mean that the urge was very weak. Number 7 would mean that the urge was one of the strongest ones that you have ever felt. If the urge was somewhere in the middle, then give it a number in between. If you had a passing thought about drinking or using drugs, write a 1. Write down what trigger was associated with the urge.

Drinking or Drug Use: If you drink or use drugs, under the **Drinking or Drug use** section we want you to put in some information about what you drank or what drug you used, how much, and the amount of alcohol in the drink:

1. In the column labeled **Time**, write down when you started drinking.

2. Under **Drink or Drug,** put down what you had. In the above example, Sally drank wine. You should put in whatever kind of drink or drug you had.

3. Next is the column labeled **Amount**. For *drinks*, write down how many drinks you had and what the size was for each drink. For the above example, Sally drank a 750-ml bottle of wine, which has about 25 ounces of liquid, or 5 standard drinks. Maybe in your case, you would have had a drink with vodka in it. We would like you to estimate the amount of vodka. One way to do this is to know the size of the glass and how many ounces of liquid it holds. We often tell people to measure their drinks, so they can understand how much they are drinking. For *drugs*, write down the amount you used. For example, if you smoked one marijuana cigarette, you could write down "one joint." Or if you vaped THC (marijuana), each vaping occasion could be written as "vaped THC or "Vaped weed/pot/marijuana/cannabis."

4. In the column labeled % **Alcohol**, write down the alcohol content of the drink you are having. Drinks will have this on the bottle or can.

5. In the column labeled **Trigger**, put down what the event was that led to the drinking or drug use.

Cigarettes: Write in the number of cigarettes you smoked that day (or N/A if you don't smoke).

Mood: Write down your overall mood each day. Circle a number between 1 and 7 to show how you feel. For example, if you are feeling very depressed, angry, or anxious, circle 7, which means "extremely bad/negative." If you are feeling "excellent," circle 1, as in best mood. If you are in between, pick a number that shows how you felt.

Additional Well-Being Change Goal: Circle "Yes" if you did something for your additional well-being change goal; circle "No" if you did not. And write in what the wellness behavior was (for instance, swam, jogged, worked out, or ate healthy).

Money Spent on Alcohol/Drugs: Write how much money you spent on alcohol/drugs that day.

Daily Drink or Drug Use Monitoring

Name _____

Date _____

Urges/Cravings

Time	How Strong? (1-7)	Trigger

Drinking or Drug use

Time	Drink or Drug	Amount (Drinks in ounces)	% Alcohol	Trigger

How many cigarettes did you smoke today? _____

Mood:

1   2   3   4   5   6   7

Excellent   Extremely bad/negative

Did you work on a well-being behavior today?	Yes No	How much money did you spend on alcohol or drugs today?

EXERCISE 1.3
Self-Monitoring

You should model self-monitoring responses, and then have one group member volunteer information about a typical drinking or drug use situation and have her role-play self-monitoring. Role-play problem situations and alternative responses, such as:

▨ **Question:** What if someone asks me what I am doing?

THERAPIST: *It is your choice how much you share with anyone. You can politely say, for instance, "I'm jotting down a note about something I want to remember." Or you can say, for instance, that you are tracking your drinking or drug use, or you could say something like, "I am on a diet" or "I am tracking wellness activities."*

▨ **Question:** This is an abstinence program. What happens if I drink or use drugs?

THERAPIST: *This treatment program does not encourage drinking or drug use. However, we want group members to be honest in their monitoring so that we can help you learn how to abstain in situations that are difficult for you. We will not discharge you from the group for reporting alcohol or drug use that week, unless we believe a higher level of care is needed—in which case you would be welcome to resume group when the inpatient care is over.*

Stress the fact that self-monitoring has been found to increase self-awareness and its important role in self-control. Self-monitoring is also part of treatment—that is, becoming aware of chains of triggers, behaviors, and consequences that were hidden before.

Abstinence Plan for Women Still Drinking or Using Drugs and/or Other Possible Problem Areas (only discuss problem areas if clients bring them up) (20 minutes)

> **Therapist Note**
> *If any client in the group is highly ambivalent about an abstinence plan because she wants to try moderated drinking, follow the suggested discussion in* Chapter 4.

Rationale:

The first step in treatment is helping you to actually stop drinking or using drugs. Then we will move on, throughout the treatment, to teaching you skills to stay sober, prevent relapse, cope better with problems, etc. Let's talk about the first step.

There are several options for stopping your use of alcohol or drugs. The general rule is that we want everyone to be shooting for abstinence in 2 weeks. Let me review the options and then we can discuss the most reasonable abstinence plan for each group member.

Boxes 1.1 to 1.4 provide a brief summary of each option for stopping alcohol or drug use. You should go through the options and briefly suggest/give feedback to each group member about what abstinence plan would be best for her. Emphasize that each group member who is not yet abstinent and is drinking with regular frequency should make an appointment with a physician who has expertise treating addiction to confirm the safest abstinence plan.

1. *One option is **inpatient alcohol detoxification**. This means that you would go to a hospital detoxification unit and stay there for about 3 to 7 days. Some detox programs provide support and monitor you, but give no medications. Hospital programs usually give you some medicine during this time to relieve withdrawal symptoms, since in this case you would be stopping "cold turkey." The advantage of an inpatient detox is that you are medically supervised, you will avoid most withdrawal symptoms if you are medicated, and it's a quick way to get the alcohol or drugs out of your system and "start fresh" in this program as your aftercare. The group will help you stay clean and prevent relapse after detox. The disadvantage to inpatient detox is that some people don't want to stay in a detox unit for a few days, and some people don't have insurance to cover this, although there are publicly funded detox programs.*

I strongly recommend inpatient detox for clients who are very heavy daily or almost-daily drinkers or drug users, who I think won't be able to stop on their own, and who are at risk for medical complications in withdrawal (personal or family history of seizures, stroke, high blood pressure, cardiac problems, etc.). To achieve abstinence from **opiates, benzodiazepines, methamphetamine,** *and some other drugs, we very strongly recommend inpatient detoxification before starting this group. Withdrawal from these drugs requires medication-assisted treatment (MAT) and medical supervision.*

2. *Another option is* **outpatient alcohol detoxification.** *This is where you would go see a physician who specializes in outpatient detoxification. Each physician may do an outpatient detox in their own way; most tend to prescribe enough medication to last a couple of days, and then have you come back to see them so they can evaluate you and determine whether they need to prescribe more medication for a few more days, depending on the severity of your withdrawal symptoms. The advantage to an outpatient detoxification is that, similar to inpatient detoxification, you get it over with quickly—typically within a week you have stopped using and passed through the initial more severe withdrawal symptoms with medication to help ease them. Another advantage is that you are under a physician's care, in case there are medical complications. A disadvantage to outpatient detox is that you must not drink alcohol while you are taking the medication the physician prescribes, and some clients end up using both, which is extremely dangerous. Also,* **outpatient alcohol detoxification options are very difficult to find—not many physicians or programs offer this option.** *Outpatient detoxification can be done using medication-assisted treatment (MAT) for* **opiates,** *and for* **benzodiazepines** *a months-long very gradual taper. These are also difficult options to find, and generally inpatient detoxification is highly recommended or required for non-alcohol drugs.*

3. *A third option is for you to* **stop drinking on your own, "cold turkey."** *I might recommend this option for people who drink episodically rather than daily, who have no history of withdrawal symptoms when they stopped in the past, who are not at risk medically (high blood pressure, history of stroke, etc.), and who are not extremely heavy drinkers. For heavy, regular drinkers or drug users, stopping "cold turkey" with no medical supervision can result in uncomfortable and/or dangerous withdrawal symptoms, and, at worst, serious and possibly fatal medical complications such as seizures. Also, withdrawal symptoms are often triggers for relapse.* **For non-alcohol drugs such as opiates and stimulants, "cold turkey" is not recommended because of the major withdrawal symptoms**

associated with these drugs. For benzodiazepines, "cold turkey" is contraindicated (that is, NOT recommended) because of major withdrawal symptoms that can be fatal.

4. *A fourth option for certain individuals is to **wind down yourself, with my guidance and with the assistance/consultation of an addiction psychiatrist.** That is, we would work together and agree on a schedule for you to gradually reduce your use of alcohol or certain drugs (like marijuana or stimulants), usually over 1 to 3 weeks. We would set a quit date that is as soon as possible without risking major withdrawal symptoms, and set up a schedule for you to gradually reduce use toward zero on that date. So, for instance, we will take out a calendar and plan for how much you can drink each day, and we'll make sure that it is always either a plateau or a reduction from one day to the next—otherwise you'll have withdrawal symptoms if you cut back a lot one day and then use more the next, and you'll have to go through withdrawal all over again. The advantage to this method is that you don't have to go to a hospital. It is gradual, so you will likely be able to avoid major withdrawal symptoms, but you must be prepared to experience some withdrawal problems, and if withdrawal symptoms escalate at any time, you will need to seek medical care as soon as possible. A disadvantage of this approach is that since it is gradual, it does take some time, and some people feel that they would rather just get it over with quickly than spread out the reduction and associated withdrawal symptoms over 1 to 3 weeks. Another disadvantage is that this approach takes a lot of planning and willpower on your part, especially in the beginning. An addiction psychiatrist or primary care provider can prescribe anti-craving medications to help. Winding down without medical supervision is NOT an option for opiate or benzodiazepine users.*

You should now briefly construct an abstinence plan for each woman in a round robin format. First, ask for questions regarding the different options of abstinence. Then, say:

Let's figure out what is the most reasonable plan for each of you, based on how much you are drinking or what your drug use is like and how often. I have a good sense of your drinking/drug use patterns that you reported during our initial intake appointment, and I will need to know if there has been a change since the last time I saw you in your drinking or drug use to help each of you decide on the best option.

Go around the room and see who is still drinking or using drugs and have them update you on the quantity/frequency pattern for the past week if anyone says their drinking or drug use pattern has changed. Now, go around and discuss, in a collaborative manner, an abstinence plan for each woman. Remember, you are the expert on this. Have each woman write it down on her Worksheet 1.1: Abstinence Plan in her workbook. This worksheet can be found near the end of Session 1 in this Therapist Guide and on Client Workbook; it can also be accessed by searching for this book's title on the Oxford Academic platform, at academic.oup.com.

For those of you who are still drinking or using daily or almost daily and choose a wind-down method, we find that the best way to reach abstinence is to first cut down quantity (that is, the amount you are drinking or using each day). Your quantity should be in a downward pattern, not down and up; that is, once you cut down to a certain amount per day, then you should not go beyond that amount going forward. Then, when you have reached a daily quantity of approximately 2 or 3 standard drinks per day, cut down frequency (that is, put in some abstinence days, plan for more and more abstinence days until you have no drinking days after the quit date), and continue to also reduce quantity. For those of you who are not drinking daily or who drink episodically (on occasion), cold turkey might be the best option for you. Of course, if you are ready to quit now, if you are at minimal risk of withdrawal, then I encourage you to begin that journey now.

Now ask for someone to volunteer whether winding down would be good for them. Suggest a way to cut down on daily drinking or drug use that minimizes withdrawal symptoms. Then, go around the room for each group member who wants to cut down gradually and briefly help them decide how much to cut down each day, based on their recent quantity/frequency of use. Have the members fill out their Worksheet 1.1: Abstinence Plan, including what the plan is and how much they should cut down (if winding down) or whether they are doing cold turkey.

Let's figure out how much each of you should cut down daily to reach your goal of abstinence.

Box 1.1. Inpatient Detoxification

- 3- to 7-day hospital stay
- Medication for withdrawal

Advantages

- Medically supervised
- Quick way to start fresh

Disadvantages

- Away from home
- May need insurance coverage

STRONGLY RECOMMENDED for

- Very heavy daily drinkers or drug users
- Those who probably can't stop otherwise
- Those at risk for medical complications
- Those using opiates or benzodiazepines

Box 1.2. Outpatient Detoxification

- Outpatient physician visits
- Limited medication for withdrawal

Advantages

- Able to stay at home
- Daily routine less disrupted

Disadvantages

- Extreme danger of taking prescribed medication and alcohol together
- Outpatient detox option very difficult to find, not typically offered

RECOMMENDED for

- Those who refuse inpatient care

Box 1.3. On One's Own: "Cold Turkey"

SHOULD MEET ALL CRITERIA:

- Drink or use drugs episodically, not daily
- Don't drink or use heavily
- No history of withdrawal symptoms
- Not at risk for medical complications

Advantages

- Quick
- No use of medication

Disadvantages

- Can result in uncomfortable or dangerous withdrawal symptoms
- Not medically supervised in case of complications
- Withdrawal symptoms can trigger relapses
- NOT recommended for users of opiates, benzodiazepines, or simulants

---

Box 1.4. Wind Down to Quit Date with Help

- Set a quit date within 1 to 3 weeks
- Agree on schedule of gradual reduction
- Reduce quantity per day first, then reduce frequency of drinking days
- Always drink/use less or same amount, not more than previous days

Advantages

- Gradual, so withdrawal lessened
- Don't need to go to a detox program
- Doesn't have same risks as "cold turkey"

Disadvantages

- Takes days to a few weeks
- Can still experience withdrawal symptoms

WORKSHEET 1.1
Abstinence Plan

My basic plan:

_____

_____

_____

When will I start my plan?

_____

_____

_____

If I'm going to get help, where will I go, or who will I call?

_____

_____

_____

If I am going to cut down gradually, how much will I cut down each day (write days and how much drinking each day to quit date)? What is my target quit date to be abstinent?

_____

_____

_____

_____

_____

Possible Problem Areas

- Self-monitoring issues: Discussed above under the introduction to self-monitoring and in Handouts 1.11 to 1.13.
- Willpower versus self-control: Some clients believe that all they need is "willpower" in order to change. They also may feel bad about themselves because they think that they don't have enough willpower. You may address this as follows:

Many people think that changing an alcohol or drug problem is just a matter of having enough willpower. I think about change differently. You definitely needed a strong will to recognize that your drinking/drug use is a problem and to decide to seek help. But successful change also requires a whole toolbox of skills—these skills give you **ways** *to carry out your* **will.** *The group sessions will introduce you to tools that will help you change successfully. The challenge for you is to try to apply these skills in your everyday lives to cope with triggers for using and to deal with cravings. Some people find their cravings are so strong that it is difficult for them to use new skills. There are anti-craving medications available to help you if you find your cravings are too overwhelming.*

- **Question:** What if I start drinking or using drugs?

THERAPIST: *Breaking a problem drinking or drug use habit is a difficult undertaking that requires a commitment to change. This treatment program is designed to help you become and stay abstinent, teaching you skills to be successful. If you feel that you are losing control or are about to drink, the rule of thumb is to leave fast, then use a behavior chain (you'll learn more about this in Session 2) and your self-monitoring to analyze your thoughts/urges. Later on, we'll talk a lot about handling slips and relapses—there is a lot more information in your workbook in Sessions 10 and 11.*

Therapist Note

It is important to communicate the fact that the treatment goal is abstinence, but that "slips" do not equal treatment failure. Remember, the client can always call her therapist before drinking or using. It will be important for you to convey a nonjudgmental attitude and openness when discussing drinking or drug use. If the client can discuss her drinking or drug use freely, then appropriate interventions can be implemented.

- **Question:** Should I go to Alcoholic Anonymous (AA)/Narcotics Anonymous (NA) meetings?

THERAPIST: *If you are already going to Twelve Step meetings, continue to go if you find it helpful. Although not a focus of our treatment, some individuals find these meetings helpful. We usually recommend that clients try a few Twelve Step meetings to see if they might be another helpful tool as a way to manage triggers or cravings. There are other "self-help" meetings for addiction that might be helpful as well, such as Smart Recovery which provides a mix of peer support and coping skills.*

- **Question:** Should I tell my kids I'm an alcoholic or a drug addict?

THERAPIST: *That's a complicated issue and one we should spend some time discussing as we go along. The answer to that question really depends on your situation; how old your kids are; and whether they've seen you drink or use drugs, have expressed concern, and so on. Generally, children ask what they need to know, and a good rule of thumb is to tell them not much more than what they ask. Also, the terms "alcoholic" and "drug addict" are not informative. We prefer to say "drink too much or use drugs" or "have an alcohol or drug problem."*

Farewell to Members Leaving the Group (10 minutes)

Have members who are leaving identify the skills they think have been most important to the changes that they have made during therapy— that is, those skills they will continue to try to implement in order to maintain their progress. Remind group members that relapses most often occur in the types of situations they are now prepared to handle.

For women finishing the group, ask them how they feel about finishing the treatment program. Explore termination issues—fear, relief, loss. Discuss referrals for additional treatment if necessary. Discuss the possibility that group members may wish to stay in contact and provide support to one another.

Each group member who is finishing treatment should also be asked to go around the room and say something positive or constructive to each of her fellow group members. These statements could focus on positive changes or steps the leaving group member has seen each of the other women make during treatment, or ways in which the leaving group member feels she herself has learned or benefited from other women in the group. Other group members also should be encouraged to give some positive feedback to the woman who is finishing treatment. Women who are finishing treatment and the therapist may also want to say something to one another.

Anticipating High-Risk Situations This Week (15 minutes)

To initiate this discussion, use Worksheet 1.2: High-Risk Situations. This worksheet can be found near the end of Session 1 in this Therapist Guide and in every session in the client workbook; it can also be accessed by searching for this book's title on the Oxford Academic platform, at academic.oup.com.

To introduce the topic, you could say:

At the end of each session, we will spend a bit of time discussing any problem situations that you think might come up around drinking/drug use over the upcoming week. As you progress through therapy, you will get better and better at anticipating and handling these. A "high-risk situation" is a situation in which you would find it very difficult not to drink or use drugs. Today, I'd like us to spend a few minutes together thinking about the upcoming week.

EXERCISE 1.4
High-Risk Situations

You should walk the group through Handout 1.14: High-Risk Situations: Sample, and elicit discussion/questions:

The idea is to complete one of these forms at the beginning of each week, perhaps on a Sunday evening as you take a look at your schedule for the upcoming week. There is a blank High-Risk Situations worksheet at the end of every session in your workbook, as this is supposed to be a weekly exercise that you continue to do each week.

Then, ask for a group member volunteer to complete her High-Risk Situations worksheet with you for her upcoming week, using the worksheet and writing her responses on the flipchart/whiteboard/blackboard. You should help her identify situations coming up this week that may be triggers for her to drink/use drugs and write down ideas to manage those triggers/high-risk situations without drinking or using drugs. Enlist support and ideas from other group members to help the volunteer complete her worksheet, as each member also jots down some of her own high-risk situations and ideas to cope with them on her own worksheet. Then, open the discussion to ask each member of the group to identify at least one high-risk situation coming up in the next week. Then, ask each woman to write on her worksheet how to handle this situation.

Also, for homework ask clients (1) to write down on the back of their self-monitoring cards how they actually handled the anticipated situation (if/when it does arise) during the week, (2) to write down any other situations that were not anticipated, and (3) to bring these cards to session for discussion next week.

Therapist Note

Make sure to point out that high-risk situations aren't always parties or special events. For a woman who drinks daily while preparing dinner, for example, that time of day should be listed as an upcoming high-risk situation this week. Most high-risk situations are embedded in our day-to-day lives, and these are just as difficult—if not more difficult—to negotiate as things like weddings and parties, at least in the beginning of therapy. Such situations get easier over time and become less and less associated with cravings to use drugs and alcohol after abstinence begins.

HANDOUT 1.14
High-Risk Situations: Sample

What high-risk situations do you think you may experience this week?

Situation 1: <u>Put baby to bed, long night ahead, thoughts racing through my head, feeling restless, sad, and anxious</u>

How can you handle this situation?

a. John stays home with the kids, I go out to the gym for a couple of hours

b. Longer days now, can go outside and take a walk or do some yard work

c. Watch a movie

d. Make popcorn and a citrus seltzer for the movie

Situation 2: <u>Monday morning, on edge, worried about finances, depression creeping in</u>

How can you handle this situation?

a. Do grounding exercise I learned, stay in the present

b. Do breathing exercise I learned to control anxiety

c. Get up, get out of my head and go about my routine

d. Call Katie and talk to her about my worries

Situation 3: <u>Picnic on Saturday with some friends and their families</u>

How can you handle this situation?

a. Bring my own soda or other non-alcoholic drink

b. Don't go if I think will be too difficult. Do something else fun with John and the kids.

c. Get to the picnic late and leave early if not doing well

d. Focus on the food and company

Worksheet 1.2
High-Risk Situations

What high-risk situations do you think you may experience this week?

Situation 1: _____

How can you handle this situation?

a. _____

b. _____

c. _____

d. _____

Situation 2: _____

How can you handle this situation?

a. _____

b. _____

c. _____

d. _____

Situation 3: _____

How can you handle this situation?

a. _____

b. _____

c. _____

d. _____

Situation 4: _____

How can you handle this situation?

a. _____

b. _____

c. _____

d. _____

Assign Homework (5 minutes)

Here is a list of homework assignments for each group member to complete between today's session and the next. Remind the women how important it is to complete the homework.

1. Complete one self-monitoring card each day.
2. On the back of your self-monitoring cards, write down high-risk situations you encountered and how you handled those that were discussed in session.
3. Read all the Session 1 material in your workbook and complete worksheets you didn't finish during the session.
4. Execute the abstinence plan.
5. If they haven't already done so, have clients make appointment with their doctors to have a physical and get blood tests for liver enzymes (including GGTP).

CHAPTER 7

Session 2: Triggers and Behavior Chains

(Corresponds to Chapter 2 in the Client Workbook)
(1.5 hours)

Notes to the Therapist Before the Session

1. For rolling-admission groups (see Chapter 3), each new member should have an individual assessment (see Chapter 5) with the group facilitator prior to joining the group. At the end of the assessment session, for women joining the group at any session (i.e., Session 2–12) after Session 1, the therapist should spend an additional 30 minutes with each new group member to provide the Client Workbook and to review basic information covered in Session 1 that the client will need to know to proceed with all subsequent sessions. This includes coverage of use of the Client Workbook and group rules, as well as a brief review of core treatment elements, including self-monitoring, psychoeducation, high-risk situations, triggers, and behavior chains (see Session 2). That way, no matter what session the new member is entering, she will be able to do daily self-monitoring and understand the basics of high-risk situations, triggers, and behavior chains.

2. Each rolling-admission group session with a new member starts with a 5-minute round robin introduction of each group member, and 10 minutes of assessment feedback to the new member(s) (see Session 1 for detailed instructions and feedback sheets). Members in the group at different stages of recovery can provide support to the new client and share their own feedback from their first session. If a new member is lacking relevant information from previous sessions, she can review sessions in the Client Workbook or you

can briefly describe the section, and/or abstinent members can be encouraged to spend time with the new member after session to explain relevant prior material.

3. For each new member entering the group in Sessions 2 to 12, follow instructions at the beginning of each session regarding Introductions and Providing Assessment Feedback in Client's First Session.

4. If this is a client's first session, you must summarize data from the pretreatment assessment to fill in a Feedback Sheet (see Handout 1.10 in Client Workbook) for each client in the group in preparation for her first session.

5. Before the session begins, write the session agenda on a flipchart, whiteboard, or blackboard.

6. If you are doing the Optional Graphing Intervention, see instructions in Chapter 3 of this Therapist Guide.

7. All worksheets and handouts used in this treatment program appear in this Therapist Guide and in the corresponding Client Workbook; worksheets (and selected handouts) can also be accessed by searching for this book's title on the Oxford Academic platform, at academic.oup.com.

Session 2 Outline

All times are approximate and should be adjusted based on clinical need and whether group time needs to be devoted to new or departing members.

1. Pre-session sign-in and substance use check (15 minutes before session begins)
2. Introductions and agenda setting (5 minutes)
3. Check-in, review of self-monitoring and homework (30 minutes)
4. Behavior chains and identifying triggers (40 minutes)
5. Farewell to members leaving the group (10 minutes)
6. Anticipating high-risk situations this week (10 minutes)
7. Assign homework (5 minutes)

1. Flipchart, whiteboard, or blackboard, felt-tip markers or chalk, eraser
2. Breathalyzer and tubes or saliva strips (optional)
3. Saliva drug tests for each group member (optional)
4. Seven self-monitoring cards for each group member (Note to therapist: Keep a stack of these to give group members at each session.)
5. OPTIONAL: Individualized graph for each woman
6. Handouts
   2.1: Graph: Alcohol/Drug Use and Urges Sample
   2.2: Behavior Chains
   2.3: The How-To of Behavior Chains
   2.4: List of Triggers—Example
   2.5: Behavior Chains: Sample—Kathy's Behavior Chains
7. Worksheets
   2.1: Graph: Alcohol/Drug Use and Urges
   2.2: List of Triggers
   2.3: Behavior Chains
   2.4: High-Risk Situations [See Client Workbook Worksheet 2.4]

Pre-Session Sign-In and Substance Use Check (15 minutes pre-session)

If any member of the group appears to be high or intoxicated, you may want to assess her blood alcohol level (BAL) with a breathalyzer or saliva strip or use a saliva drug screen. Regardless of formal testing, though, if a group member is visibly high or intoxicated, review the treatment agreement with her and then let her know that she will not be allowed to attend this session. Clients who miss a session will not receive a make-up session, but encourage them to read the handouts they missed for that session and complete the homework for the following week. You should assist the client in arranging alternate transportation home, review her abstinence plan, and remind her of her abstinence goal.

Introductions and Agenda Setting (5 minutes)

You will introduce new members joining the group this session, and provide an overview (i.e., set agenda) of what will be covered in the session and explain that the purpose of Session 2 is to: (a) review the week for alcohol/drug use; (b) review each woman's prior week triggers, alcohol and drug use, cravings, and coping strategies including what she could have done differently or can do differently going forward; (c) review tracking of well-being activities; (d) introduce use of "behavior chains" to understand and change drinking behavior/drug use (the big picture), create a personalized list of drinking/drug use triggers, and practice completing a few behavior chains; and (e) identify and brainstorm coping strategies for this week's upcoming high-risk situations for drinking/drug use. Ask the group if there is anything pressing they would like to discuss today in addition to the planned material. Note who is absent from the group today in a matter-of-fact way without saying why or giving any information about the absent member: "XX and JJ are not with us today; we hope to see them next week."

Check-In, Review of Self-Monitoring and Homework (30 minutes)

Check-in follows a "round robin" format, in which drinking status and homework are emphasized. To introduce the round robin check-in:

We're going to go around the room using what we call a "round robin check-in" to get a brief version of how your week has been, focusing on your alcohol use, drug use, cravings, and triggers; how you coped with triggers and cravings; in hindsight what you might have done differently (with therapist and group input/ideas as well); homework you completed and what was helpful about it. We also will answer or clarify any questions or concerns about the homework material. Each group member will have a few minutes [depending on how many women there are in the group] *to discuss with the group how your coping with alcohol/drug use triggers has been this week.*

Go around the room and ask each group member how her week was (focusing on alcohol and or drug use); listen while looking over her self-monitoring cards; and link what she is saying to her daily cards for alcohol/drug cravings, triggers, and use. Use information from this for specific topics in the rest of the session. Check in with each group member and discuss the progress of her abstinence plan. Update the plan if necessary. Also remember to ask each client at the end of her round robin time about what homework she was able to complete.

You should reinforce self-recording behavior, check for questions or problems, and help group members develop solutions for difficulties related to self-recording procedures. Ask members if they have any questions. Possible questions to anticipate include:

- **Question:** I thought about drinking the whole morning. Is that one urge or more than one?

THERAPIST: *You had the urge continually?*

CLIENT: Not every minute.

THERAPIST: *Well, each time you have a thought or an image about having a specific type of drink or a drink in a particular situation, that counts as a separate urge. Can you share some specific situations you thought about?*

- **Question:** Why are my urges so much higher than everyone else's? Why am I the only one still drinking?

THERAPIST: *It's natural that you would want to compare your drinking/ drug use and urges to those of the other group members. Although this can be an important motivator, it also is important to remember that everyone has her own unique path to abstinence. You're working on it, so be patient with yourself, and think of the changes you've already made! What does the group think about what _____ said?*

Optional Graphing Intervention for Outpatient Treatment Settings

See the detailed instructions in Chapter 3 of this guide for how to use the graphs located here in Session 2 of the Therapist Guide and in the Client Workbook (Handout 2.1. Graph: Alcohol/Drug Use and Urges Sample and Worksheet 2.1. Graph: Alcohol/Drug Use and Urges). This intervention will allow each woman to track her progress by entering weekly data summarized from her daily monitoring cards: 1. Number of drinks; 2. Number of drugs used; 3. Number of urges/cravings; and 4. Average strength of urges/cravings.

Other Homework Review .

Review all other homework clients did during the prior week. Reinforce clients for completing homework and discuss barriers experienced in completing the homework. Ask questions such as, *"What did you learn from the homework?"* or *"How can you use the homework to help you in the future?"*

Remember that as part of homework review, each week you need to review group members' recording of high-risk situations and how these were handled: *"Who wants to share how you handled one of your high-risk situations this week without drinking/using drugs?"* Elicit high-risk examples from two or three group members and get feedback from other members. Remember to have group members direct their comments to the other group members, and not just to you. Point out common types of high-risk situations among the group members and encourage women facing similar situations to share how they coped or ideas for coping. Selectively model and re- peat empowering and motivational positive affirmations that group members give to one another: for example, *"We know this is hard, you're doing great." "Next time you'll be able to use a different strategy, hang in there."*

Also, ask about progress with doctor's appointments and blood tests. Due to time constraints, group members should discuss any concerns about their blood test or feedback with you after the group. Ask each client to bring in a copy of her lab results and give it to you. You can give feedback to the client during review of homework either that week or the week after.

Therapist Note

You should manage participation so that there is enough time to go around the room in a round robin fashion and give each group member a chance to speak. Keep in mind that 10 to 30 minutes total is allotted for check-in depending on how many women are in the group. If homework is not done, you should ask what made it difficult for the client to complete the homework. The importance of completing homework should be discussed, and a firm commitment for the future should be stressed in a nonjudgmental way.

Share the following with the group:

The time in the treatment group is only part of the process. The real change occurs when you practice changing your lives in the real world. The group will help you get ideas, stay motivated, keep you on track, and develop an understanding of the problem. But actually changing behavior takes place in your everyday life—at home, at work, with family, friends, and so on.

Therapist Note

The following are some tips for managing members' participation to maintain the temporal structure of the session. For habitually quiet members or those who appear upset or distressed, you should acknowledge them with empathic nonverbal behavior, but do not call on them to elicit participation right away, except during their turn in the round robin. Look for opportunities to invite limited participation of habitually quiet members to help them become comfortable

---

sharing. Frequently ask the group for their feedback on particular group members' contributions, to set up the expectation that group members will be doing a lot of the work in the room. Everyone in the group learns by hearing the experiences and advice of others. Model and facilitate a tone of supportive, constructive, and compassionate feedback in the group. Don't be confrontational, but also don't condone or reassure a woman about her drinking/drug use or lack of work outside the group sessions. For instance, <u>don't</u> say, "It's okay, you had a really hard week; of course you drank a bit." Say instead, "You certainly had a hard week! In hindsight, what could you have done differently in response to trigger xxx?"

Group members who are having substantial difficulty with their abstinence plan or who appear to be at risk for an emergency should be asked discreetly to remain after group for an individual check-in with you.

Graph: Alcohol/Drug Use and Urges Sample

Number of urges

Number of drinks

Average intensity of urges

54

48

42

36

30

24

18

12

6

Baseline

1   2   3   4   5   6   7   8   9   10   11   12

Week

WORKSHEET 2.1

Graph: Alcohol/Drug Use and Urges

Week

Baseline

1 2 3 4 5 6 7 8 9 10 11 12

Rationale: Explain to the group that learning to identify situations that trigger drinking or drug use and learning to cope with them will help group members find it easier to stay sober/clean. Behavior chains (habit analysis) should be discussed as the first step in understanding and gaining self-control over problematic drinking or drug use. Tell the group that problem drinking or drug use is a habit in response to specific triggers and the habit is maintained by both short-term and long-term consequences. Use Handout 2.2: Behavior Chains and Handout 2.3: The How-To's of Behavior Chains, and explain the following using illustrations on the flip chart.

You can follow along in your workbook, Handout 2.2: Behavior Chains. The first step in achieving abstinence is understanding more about your drinking/drug use. Together, we're going to look at situations that are triggers for you (i.e., situations that are high risks for you to drink or use drugs) and how you react to them. This is called a **behavior chain.** *Then, in future sessions, we will try to come up with a plan to manage each situation that will work for you. A behavior chain can be broken down into the following steps:*

1. *Events (cues, or triggers) that come before drinking/drug use*
2. *Thoughts and feelings that come before drinking/drug use*
3. *Your behavior (i.e., how many drinks or what drugs consumed, your estimated blood alcohol level) in response to those events*
4. *What happens during or just after drinking/drug use (short-term consequences, which often are positive)*
5. *What happens later after drinking/drug use (long-term consequences, which often are negative)*

Ask the group to turn to Handouts 2.2 and 2.3 in their workbooks. Using the handouts, explain the behavior chains to the group.

HANDOUT 2.2
Behavior Chains

A behavior chain is a very important part of this treatment. A behavior chain involves looking at what happens before, during, and after a drinking or drug use episode. This helps us learn about the chains of events that keep drinking or drug use going.

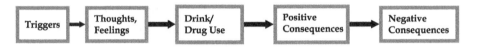

Every chain follows a pattern. Triggers lead to thoughts and feelings that set up the drinker/user. After drinking or using drugs, some good things happen (positive consequences) immediately, and bad things (negative consequences) come later. Let's look at each step of the chain.

Triggers	People, places, and things are associated with drinking or drug use. A trigger is something that occurs before drinking/drug use. A trigger can be something easy to see or something sneaky. Often the drinker/user is not aware of the triggers. Triggers don't directly make people drink or use drugs; they just set up thoughts and feelings connected to drinking/using.
Thoughts, Feelings	The triggers bring up thoughts and feelings that are connected to drinking/using. These thoughts and feelings can be nice or unpleasant. Some examples are "I feel so anxious, I need to drink to be more sociable," or "I'm in a great mood now, it will be even better with some weed," or "A drink will help me relax."
Drink/Drug Use	Drinking or using drugs is something you do. It is a behavior that is a part of the chain. Calculate exactly how many standard drinks you had and what your estimated blood alcohol level was, or how much of a drug you used.
Positive Consequences	Very often something nice happens when someone drinks/uses. For instance, a feeling of relaxation happens quickly after drinking or using certain drugs. Such positive consequences usually happen in the short term—that is, while drinking or using. That's why people keep drinking/using: because there's usually an immediate positive effect of alcohol or drugs, such as euphoria or relaxation.
Negative Consequences	The trouble that comes with alcohol and drug use often comes later. The trouble comes in many forms: hangover, headache, irregular heartbeat, eating too much while high, "drunk dialing," blackouts, embarrassing behavior, family arguments, problems with a boss, poor health, etc. Because the trouble comes later on, people don't always make the connection between the trouble and their drinking/using. Many times, the possible trouble is out of mind when thoughts of the pleasant parts of drinking or using are on your mind.
	Also, one important short-term negative consequence of drinking/drug use is that judgment is impaired *after only one drink or use of a drug*, which makes it very difficult to stop at one or two drinks. And, drinking or using ignite the "reward center" of your brain—that is, it ignites craving for more, which reduces ability to stop at just one or two.

The first part of therapy is to construct behavior chains of what starts and keeps you drinking. Let's find out about your triggers. Later, we will learn ways to break the chains.

For example, say you had an argument with your partner in the evening and you think: "I need to relax! A couple of drinks will relieve my stress." You go over to your friend's house and you end up having more than a few. You get a DWI (driving while intoxicated) on the way home, and the next morning you cannot get up and are late for work.

In this example, **first**, having an argument with your partner and feeling tense happened before you drank and "set the stage" for drinking. We call these "triggers"—risky situations, places, people, times, or feelings that lead up to your drinking. Triggers are like amber or red traffic lights; they signal "Danger—trouble coming up ahead unless you stop." **Second**, triggers are usually associated with certain thoughts and feelings. Feelings in the above example would be tension, anger, and anticipation of relaxing. Examples of thoughts are "I need to unwind, forget my troubles, lift depression, wash away anger." **Third**, starting to drink, but then not being able to stop at two or three drinks. **Fourth**, feeling the positive consequences of drinking, which usually are immediate, such as feeling relaxed. These things are also important and go on during or after drinking itself. **Fifth**, not being able to get up and being late for work are more long-term consequences of drinking; they happen as a result of drinking. These are mostly negative consequences.

This whole series of events is called a <u>Behavior Chain, in which the behavior is drinking or drug use. It</u> <u>is a chain of events</u>—triggers, drinking behaviors, and consequences—that you can learn to interrupt.

Trigger	Thoughts, Feelings	Drink/Drug (When/Where?)	Positive Consequences	Negative Consequences
Argument with my partner	◆ He won't listen to me. ◆ I am really angry. ◆ I feel tense. ◆ Some wine will calm my nerves. ◆ I'll just have a glass of wine.	◆ At my friend's house for 2 hours—had six 5-ounce glasses of wine (6 standard drinks) ◆ Estimated blood alcohol level = .11	◆ Feeling relaxed, sociable, and happy for 3 hours ◆ Temporarily don't care about anger at partner	◆ Lost control over drinking— drank more than intended ◆ DWI on way home ◆ Less empowered in relationship ◆ Guilt, shame ◆ Worse marital problems

1. Write in the drink/drug column when and where the drinking or drug use happened. In our example, the person had six, 5-ounce glasses of wine (i.e., six standard drinks) at her girlfriend's place.

2. Think back to what happened before the drinking or drug use happened. What were the people, places, or things that set up the drinking/use? Write these things in the trigger column. In this example, the person had an argument with her partner and was still upset.

3. After writing the triggers, think back to those thoughts and feelings that made drinking/using more likely. In this example, the person thinks about calming her nerves with some wine. She may have thought that one or two drinks would not hurt anyone.

4. Think about what happened after drinking/using. Remember the good things, the positive consequences. It is realistic to say that good things will happen, in the short term, to people when they drink/use. In our example, the person feels more sociable and happier.

5. Now think about the things that happened later: the negative consequences. The problems created by drinking often come later on. In this example, our person got a DWI (driving while intoxicated) charge.

As with most people, the person in our example falls into a pattern. Some triggers will set off thoughts and emotions that lead to drinking/using. The drinking/using leads to some nice things happening, and also to lack of judgment and to more impulsivity. These nice things, lack of judgment, and lack of inhibition encourage the drinker/user to keep using.

The behavior chain helps us learn about these kinds of patterns. Most people are not aware of the patterns and habits that happen in their lives, and it takes some detective work to identify these patterns.

Now it is your turn. On your Worksheet 2.3: Behavior Chains, you will fill out the pattern that happened the last few times you drank or used. Put down as many details as you can remember. The goal here is to learn from the past so that we can make changes for the future.

Continue with the session as follows:

We will look at each part of the chain and find out what your patterns are and how to change them. Now perhaps you can begin to see why I ask such detailed questions; I need to know precisely what your particular drinking or using patterns are like. Every individual is different. This is all part of the treatment.

The first part of gaining control of your drinking/drug use will be to analyze your drinking/using habits, the second part will be to learn ways to deal with triggers, the third part will be to learn positive alternatives to alcohol or drug use (give examples of assertion or lifestyle balance), *and the fourth part will be to learn how to maintain these changes.*

By understanding your behavior chains for drinking/using, you are taking the next step to feeling in charge. Instead of being at the mercy of your triggers, you will be able to take control, to analyze the situation and figure out how to deal with each trigger instead of just reacting *to it by drinking or using. Also, the idea is to take a moment in response to a trigger or craving and think through the chain to the negative consequences if you drink/use drugs; then you can use that awareness to loop back to how you choose to respond to the trigger: drink/use drugs, or do something different.*

The choice to suffer or not to suffer negative consequences of drinking/using will be yours!

EXERCISE 2.1
List of Triggers

In this exercise, the clients will start developing some of their own behavior chains by first thinking more about their triggers. For this exercise, they will be using Handout 2.4: List of Triggers—Example and Worksheet 2.2: List of Triggers.

Therapist Note

Work with one group member volunteer to construct her list of triggers (Worksheet 2.2) on the flipchart (you will fill in the trigger list as you and the client come up with triggers, while other group members watch and offer suggestions, if appropriate).

Let's construct a trigger list together for one person here, so you can all see how it's done. Then, we will have some time to open up the discussion to help everyone fill in some of their own list of triggers together. Who wants to volunteer?

Therapist Note

You will stand at the flipchart and fill in a list of triggers with the volunteer, who will remain in her seat and talk through the triggers with you. EMPHASIZE THAT THE MORE SPECIFIC THE TRIGGERS, THE BETTER. That is, rather than just "restaurant," ask, "In which specific restaurants do you most often want to order a glass of wine with dinner?" and then write down the names of those restaurants. Or, instead of "time of day," ask, "You mentioned that you pour your first glass of wine when you start making dinner. What time is that usually?" and write down "5 pm weeknights" and also write "cooking dinner," and "is it also fair to write kitchen at 5 pm weeknights as a trigger for you?" Rather than "friends," ask, "Who specifically do you drink with?" Write specific first names: "Lisa, Joyce, Heather, Joe, and Susanne."

Let's start creating a list of all of your triggers. (Use Handout 2.4: List of Triggers—Example and Worksheet 2.2: List of Triggers). As you can see on the handout, triggers can be environmental, interpersonal, emotional, and so on. There's an example with some common triggers for women.

After discussing/writing down some triggers in each category, elicit other group members' input:

Can anyone think of any other triggers for _____'s drinking/drug use that we might have missed based on what you know so far about her drinking pattern and history?

Individual Component of Exercise 2.1

You will then open up the discussion to work together as a group for members to list their triggers on their worksheets, eliciting their own ideas and also from what you know from self-recording cards, intake information, and discussion thus far about each woman's triggers.

Now, let's take some time for each group member to work on your own trigger worksheet. Use Handout 2.4 in your workbook. While we're doing that, share out loud and let's discuss what you're thinking and writing.

Generate some discussion about triggers that group members are mentioning and writing down. Then ask: *What sort of triggers did you generate for your list?* (Discuss some triggers, point out others you may have noticed as possibly important, and give suggestions for making them as specific as possible.) *Good—great job. This week, for homework, you can spend some time filling in your trigger worksheet and then we can all discuss what you came up with at the beginning of next week's session.*

HANDOUT 2.4
List of Triggers—Example

Environmental
(places, things)

5 pm on weeknight, in kitchen preparing dinner at home

Saturday evening

Restaurant (Rosie's Italian, or Center Stage Steak)

Messy house

Dinner party or barbecue

10 pm, home alone

Interpersonal
(people)

Eating out with John (husband)—anywhere but the diner

Night out with the girlfriends (Lisa, Joyce, Heather)—bar, dinner, club

Other waitresses, after work (leftover wine)

When my mother is bossy

Argument with John

Kids are loud and boisterous when I'm tired

Emotions/Thoughts

Anxiety

Depression, sadness

Anger, frustration

Loneliness

Stressed out, tense

Physical

PMS

Menstrual cramps

Can't sleep

Hot flashes

Chronic pain flare-up from shoulder injury

Environmental
(places, things)

_____

_____

_____

_____

_____

Interpersonal
(people)

_____

_____

_____

_____

Emotions/Thoughts

_____

_____

_____

_____

_____

Physical

_____

_____

_____

_____

EXERCISE 2.2
Behavior Chains

For this exercise, you and the clients will need Handout 2.5: Behavior Chains: Sample—Kathy's Behavior Chains and Worksheet 2.3: Behavior Chains. You will walk the group through the sample behavior chain and then ask for a volunteer to map out a personalized behavior chain together with you while the rest of group watches and discusses.

> *Now we will use our trigger worksheet to pick out a trigger and do a behavior chain for that trigger, as we described before* [point to flipchart]. *Let's run through one together to show you how, and then you'll each work out one here on your own. Who would like to volunteer to work out a behavior chain with me?*

> [To volunteer:] *There is an example of a completed behavior chain (Handout 2.5) in the Client Workbook. This is a typical chain of events for many women who we've treated.* [Walk volunteer and group through the example.] *Now, let's take one of your triggers and work it through. Which would you like to use?* [Work through a behavior chain with the volunteer using Worksheet 2.3: Behavior Chains; the group participates by offering input and suggestions.] *Good. How was it to do this chain? What did you learn?*

When you and the volunteer have worked through one behavior chain, ask the group how they felt about doing it, what stood out, and any surprise reactions. Then ask each woman to work on her own behavior chain for a real situation that she has experienced, with open discussion during so they can share with the group what they're coming up with. Do not have the group work in silence for 5 minutes and then ask how it went. Rather, this should be each group member working on her own personal chain using Worksheet 2.3: Behavior Chains, with concurrent group discussion going on about what they are writing. Help clients understand the various parts of the drinking chain triggers and consequences, and encourage them to be specific: How many standard drinks did you have in that situation? What do you think your estimated blood alcohol level was? Point out that there are both positive and negative consequences (give examples).

You should assign homework for group members to work out one more behavior chain of a real situation they experienced when they were drinking/using, and to work out a second behavior chain of the same trigger putting in a non-drinking/using alternative behavior they could have made in response to the same trigger and thoughts and feelings, thinking through what the positive and negative consequences of the non-drinking/using response might have been.

HANDOUT 2.5

Behavior Chains: Sample—Kathy's Behavior Chains

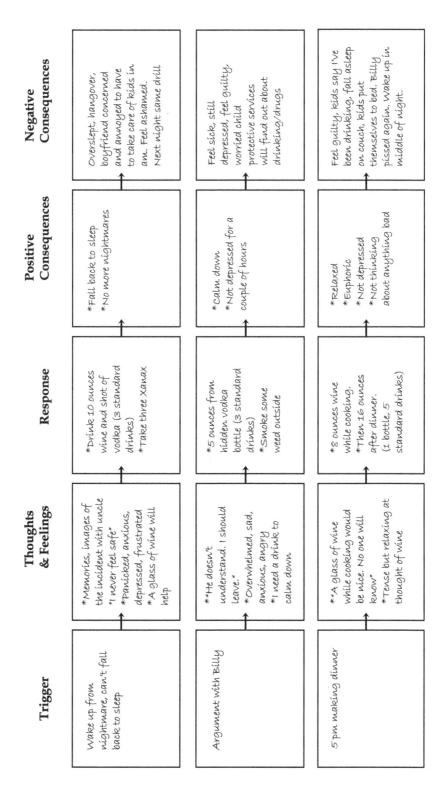

Trigger	Thoughts & Feelings	Response	Positive Consequences	Negative Consequences
Wake up from nightmare, can't fall back to sleep	*Memories, images of the incident with uncle "I never feel safe" *Panicked, anxious, depressed, frustrated *A glass of wine will help	*Drink 10 ounces wine and shot of vodka (3 standard drinks) *Take three Xanax	*Fall back to sleep *No more nightmares	Overslept, hangover, boyfriend concerned and annoyed to have to take care of kids in am. Feel ashamed. Next night same drill
Argument with Billy	"He doesn't understand. I should leave." *Overwhelmed, sad, anxious, angry *I need a drink to calm down	*5 ounces from hidden vodka bottle (3 standard drinks) *Smoke some weed outside	*Calm down *Not depressed for a couple of hours	Feel sick, still depressed, feel guilty, worried child protective services will find out about drinking/drugs
5 pm making dinner	*"A glass of wine while cooking would be nice. No one will know." *Tense but relaxing at thought of wine	*8 ounces wine while cooking. *Then 16 ounces after dinner. (1 bottle, 5 standard drinks)	*Relaxed *Euphoric *Not depressed *Not thinking about anything bad	Feel guilty, kids say I've been drinking, fall asleep on couch, kids put themselves to bed. Billy pissed again. Wake up in middle of night.

WORKSHEET 2.3
Behavior Chains

Trigger	Thoughts & Feelings	Response	Positive Consequences	Negative Consequences
	→	→	→	→
	→	→	→	→
	→	→	→	→

Farewell to Members Leaving the Group (10 minutes)

Have members who are leaving identify the skills they think have been most important to the changes that they have made during therapy—that is, those skills they will continue to try to implement in order to maintain their progress. Remind group members that relapses most often occur in the types of situations they are now prepared to handle.

For women finishing the group, ask them how they feel about finishing the treatment program. Explore termination issues—fear, relief, loss. Discuss referrals for additional treatment if necessary. Discuss the possibility that group members may wish to stay in contact and provide support to one another.

Each group member who is finishing treatment should also be asked to go around the room and say something positive or constructive to each of her fellow group members. These statements could focus on positive changes or steps the leaving group member has seen each of the other women make during treatment, or ways in which the leaving group member feels she herself has learned or benefited from other women in the group. Other group members also should be encouraged to give some positive feedback to the woman who is finishing treatment. Women who are finishing treatment and the therapist may also want to say something to one another.

Anticipating High-Risk Situations This Week (10 minutes)

Rationale:

At the end of each session, we will spend a bit of time discussing any problem situations that each member thinks might come up around drinking or drug use this week. As you each progress through therapy, you will get better and better at anticipating and handling these. A "high-risk situation" is a situation in which you would find it very difficult not to drink. Today, I'd like us each to spend a few minutes together thinking about the upcoming week. [For each group member:] *Are there any situations that you might encounter this week that would tempt you to drink or use drugs? (See sample of a completed High Risk Situation worksheet in Session 1 of this manual, Handout 1.14).*

EXERCISE 2.3
High-Risk Situations and Executing High-Risk Situation Plans

Use Worksheet 2.4: High-Risk Situations, located in the Client Workbook:

> *Now let's each use Worksheet 2.4: High-Risk Situations to write in a high-risk situation for this upcoming week and brainstorm together about strategies/solutions you can use to cope with that high-risk situation in order to avoid drinking or using drugs in response to it. Are there any situations that you might encounter this week that would tempt you to drink or use drugs?*

Elicit examples of upcoming high-risk situations from members and brainstorm together to generate plans for how to handle the situation for two or three group members. Write ideas about how to handle this situation on the High-Risk Situations worksheet. Refer to Session 1 in this guide for a copy of the worksheet or to the Client Workbook (Worksheet 2.4) for a client version of the worksheet.

Assign Homework (5 minutes)

Here is a list of homework assignments for each group member to complete between today's session and the next. Remind the women how important it is to complete the homework.

1. Complete one self-monitoring card each day.
2. On the back of your self-monitoring cards, write down high-risk situations you encountered and how you handled them.
3. Read all the Session 2 material in your workbook and complete worksheets you didn't finish during the session.
4. Complete Worksheet 2.4: High-Risk Situations, located in the Client Workbook, and execute high-risk situation plans.

CHAPTER 8

Session 3: Presence of Heavy Drinkers/Drug Users in Social Network; Self-Management Plans

(Corresponds to Chapter 3 in the Client Workbook)

(1.5 hours)

1. For rolling-admission groups (see Chapter 3), each new member should have an individual assessment (see Chapter 5) with the group facilitator prior to joining the group. At the end of the assessment session, for women joining the group at any session (i.e., Session 2–12) after Session 1, the therapist should spend an additional 30 minutes with each new group member to provide the Client Workbook and to review basic information covered in Session 1 that the client will need to know to proceed with all subsequent sessions. This includes coverage of use of the Client Workbook and group rules, as well as a brief review of core treatment elements, including self-monitoring, psychoeducation, high-risk situations, triggers, and behavior chains (see Session 2). That way, no matter what session the new member is entering, she will be able to do daily self-monitoring and understand the basics of high-risk situations, triggers, and behavior chains.

2. Each rolling-admission group session with a new member starts with a 5-minute round robin introduction of each group member, and 10 minutes of assessment feedback to the new member(s) (see Session 1 for detailed instructions and feedback sheets). Members in the group at different stages of recovery can provide support to the new client and share their own feedback from their first session. If a new member is lacking relevant information from previous sessions,

she can review sessions in the Client Workbook or you can briefly describe the section, and/or abstinent members can be encouraged to spend time with the new member after session to explain relevant prior material.

3. For each new member entering the group in Sessions 2 to 12, follow instructions at the beginning of each session regarding Introductions and Providing Assessment Feedback in Client's First Session.

4. If this is a client's first session, you must summarize data from the pretreatment assessment to fill in a Feedback Sheet (see Handout 1.10 in Client Workbook) for each client in the group in preparation for her first session.

5. Before the session begins, write the session agenda on a flipchart, whiteboard, or blackboard.

6. If you are doing the Optional Graphing Intervention, see instructions in Chapter 3 of this Therapist Guide.

7. All worksheets and handouts used in this treatment program appear in this Therapist Guide and in the corresponding Client Workbook; worksheets (and selected handouts) can also be accessed by searching for this book's title on the Oxford Academic platform, at academic. oup.com.

Session 3 Outline

All times are approximate and should be adjusted based on clinical need and whether group time needs to be devoted to new or departing members.

1. Pre-session sign-in and substance use check (15 minutes before session begins)
2. Introductions and agenda setting (5 minutes)
3. Check-in, review of self-monitoring and homework (20 minutes)
4. Presence of heavy drinkers/drug users in social network (20 minutes)
5. Self-management planning (35 minutes)
6. Farewell to members leaving the group (10 minutes)
7. Anticipating high-risk situations this week (5 minutes)
8. Assign homework (5 minutes)

Materials Needed

1. Flipchart, whiteboard, or blackboard, felt-tip markers or chalk, eraser
2. Breathalyzer and tubes or saliva strips (optional)
3. Saliva drug tests for each group member (optional)
4. Seven self-monitoring cards for each group member (Note to therapist: Keep a stack of these to give group members at each session.)
5. OPTIONAL: Individualized graph for each woman
6. Handouts

    3.1: Who's in Your Circle? Who's in Your Corner?

    3.2: Your Social Network Example

    3.3: Heavy Drinkers/Drug Users in Your Social Network: Sample

    3.4: How to Manage Triggers

    3.5: Self-Management Planning Sheet—Example 1

    3.6: Self-Management Planning Sheet—Example 2
7. Worksheets

    3.1: Behavior Chains

    3.2: Your Social Network

    3.3: Heavy Drinkers/Drug Users in Your Social Network

    3.4: Self-Management Planning

    3.5: High-Risk Situations [See Client Workbook Worksheet 3.5]

Pre-Session Sign-In and Substance Use Check (15 minutes pre-session)

If any member of the group appears to be high or intoxicated, you may want to assess her blood alcohol level (BAL) with a breathalyzer or saliva strip or use a saliva drug screen. Regardless of formal testing, though, if a group member is visibly high or intoxicated, review the treatment agreement with her and let her know that she will not be allowed to attend this session. Clients who miss a session will not receive a make-up session, but encourage them to read the handouts they missed for that session and complete the homework for the following week. You should assist the client in arranging alternate transportation home, review her abstinence plan, and remind her of her abstinence goal.

Introductions and Agenda Setting (5 minutes)

You will introduce new members joining the group this session, and provide an overview (i.e., set agenda) of what will be covered in this session: *Today we will do an exercise to assess and discuss group members' social support networks, including the presence of alcohol/drug users.* The group will also learn about "self-management plans"—brainstorming for how to deal with client triggers. Ask the group if there is anything pressing that they would like to discuss today in addition to the planned material. Note the absence of missing group members without revealing protected health information.

Check-In, Review of Self-Monitoring and Homework (20 minutes)

Check-in follows a "round robin" format, in which drinking status and homework are emphasized. To introduce the round robin check-in:

We're going to go around the room using what we call a "round robin check-in" to get a brief version of how your week has been, focusing on your alcohol use, drug use, cravings, and triggers; how you coped with triggers and cravings; in hindsight what you might have done differently (with therapist and group input/ideas as well); homework you completed and what was helpful about it. We also will answer or clarify any questions or concerns about the homework material. Each group member will have a few minutes [depending on how many women there are in the group] *to discuss with the group how your coping with alcohol/drug use triggers has been this week.*

> **Therapist Note**
> *Try to pay particular attention to women's specific themes (e.g., right to self-care, empowerment) to link experiences to the specific theme: "One theme I've heard that's common among several of you is . . ."*

Go around the room and ask each group member how her week was (focusing on alcohol and/or drug use); listen while looking over her self-monitoring cards; and link what she is saying to her daily cards for alcohol/drug cravings, triggers, and use. Use information from this for specific topics in the rest of the session. Check in with each group member and discuss the progress of her abstinence plan. Update the plan if necessary. Also remember to ask each client at the end of her round robin time about what homework she was able to complete.

You should reinforce self-recording behavior, check for questions or problems, and help group members develop solutions for difficulties related to self-recording procedures. Ask members if they have any questions. Possible questions to anticipate include:

▪ **Question:** I thought about drinking the whole morning. Is that one urge or more than one?

THERAPIST: *You had the urge continually?*

CLIENT: Not every minute.

THERAPIST: *Well, each time you have a thought or an image about having a specific type of drink or a drink in a particular situation, that counts as a separate urge. Can you share some specific situations you thought about?*

▪ **Question:** Why are my urges so much higher than everyone else's? Why am I the only one still drinking?

THERAPIST: *It's natural that you would want to compare your drinking/ drug use and urges to those of the other group members. Although this can be an important motivator, it also is important to remember that everyone has her own unique path to abstinence. You're working on it, so be patient with yourself, and think of the changes you've already made! What does the group think about what _____ said?*

Therapist Note

After reviewing the daily monitoring cards, for outpatient settings you may wish to include the optional Graphing Intervention here.

Optional Graphing Intervention for Outpatient Treatment Settings

See the detailed instructions in Chapter 3 of this guide for how to use the graphs located in Session 2 of the Therapist Guide and in the Client Workbook (Handout 2.1. Graph: Alcohol/Drug Use and Urges Sample and Worksheet 2.1. Graph: Alcohol/Drug Use and Urges). This intervention will allow each woman to track her progress by entering weekly data summarized from her daily monitoring cards: 1. Number of drinks; 2. Number of drugs used; 3. Number of urges/cravings; and 4. Average strength of urges/cravings.

Other Homework Review

Review all other homework clients did during the prior week. Reinforce clients for completing homework and discuss barriers experienced in completing the homework. Ask questions such as, *"What did you learn from the homework?"* or *"How can you use the homework to help you in the future?"*

After reviewing group members' behavior chains, ask that they complete two more behavior chains for situations that occur during the week, using Worksheet 3.1: Behavior Chains.

WORKSHEET 3.1
Behavior Chains

Trigger		Thoughts & Feelings		Response		Positive Consequences		Negative Consequences
	→		→		→		→	
	→		→		→		→	
	→		→		→		→	

Remember that as part of homework review, each week you need to review group members' recording of high-risk situations and how these were handled: *"Who wants to share how you handled one of your high-risk situations this week without drinking/using drugs?"* Elicit high-risk examples from two or three group members and get feedback from other members. Remember to have group members direct their comments to the other group members, and not just to you. Point out common types of high-risk situations among the group members and encourage women facing similar situations to share how they coped or ideas for coping. Selectively model and repeat empowering and motivational positive affirmations that group members give to one another: for example, *"We know this is hard, you're doing great." "Next time you'll be able to use a different strategy, hang in there."*

Also, ask about progress with doctor's appointments and blood tests. Due to time constraints, group members should discuss any concerns about their blood test or feedback with you after the group. Ask each client to bring in a copy of her lab results and give it to you. You can give feedback to the client during review of homework either that week or the week after.

Therapist Note

You should manage participation so that there is enough time to go around the room in a round robin fashion and give each group member a chance to speak. Keep in mind that 10 to 30 minutes total is allotted for check-in depending on how many women are in the group. If homework is not done, you should ask what made it difficult for the client to complete the homework. The importance of completing homework should be discussed, and a firm commitment for the future should be stressed in a nonjudgmental way.

Share the following with the group:

The time in the treatment group is only part of the process. The real change occurs when you practice changing your lives in the real world. The group will help you get ideas, stay motivated, keep you on track, and develop an understanding of the problem. But actually changing behavior takes place in your everyday life—at home, at work, with family, friends, and so on.

Group members who are having substantial difficulty with their abstinence plan or who appear to be at risk for an emergency should be asked discreetly to remain after group for an individual check-in with you.

Presence of Heavy Drinkers/Drug Users in Social Network (20 minutes)

Rationale:

Please follow along with Handout 3.1. We know from research on female problem drinkers and drug users that almost 50% of their spouses/partners drink or use drugs at moderate to heavy levels. We know that heavy drinkers and drug users in a woman's social network can be triggers for the woman to drink or use drugs herself. Women are more likely to drink/ use drugs when their friends do so. We want to help you learn to manage this set of triggers so that you can make your choice to stay sober whether or not other people in your social circle are drinking or using drugs. We want you to think of yourself as an independent operator, able to decide that your sobriety is a priority regardless of how other people see it.

Who's in Your Circle? Who's in Your Corner?

. . . dealing with heavy drinkers and drug users in your social network

What Is a Social Network?

A social network is your "social circle"—people who are important to you, people with whom you spend most of your time, people you care about most, people who care about you. It can include your spouse or partner, children, parents, siblings, other relatives, friends, coworkers, and so on.

Social networks are extremely important to women. Men tend to think in terms of hierarchies (who has more power), while women tend to think in terms of circles (who is in my inner circle of friends; who is more distant).

What Does a Social Network Have to Do with Drinking or Drug Use?

We hear things like: "Everyone I know drinks or uses drugs. I don't use as much as most people I know!" That's because people who drink or use drugs tend to socialize with others who also drink or use drugs. That can make it seem "normal" to drink frequently or heavily. Among 102 female problem drinkers in a recent study, the more drinkers in the social network and the more heavy drinkers in the social network, the more often the woman drank herself. Among female problem drinkers, about 42% said that their spouse/partner was a moderate or heavy drinker; 29% of their male partners had a current or prior drinking problem.

What Does Your Social Network Have to Do with Your Drinking or Drug Use?

Emotional situations and social situations are among the strongest drinking and drug use triggers for women. Partners, family members, friends, and co-workers who are heavy drinkers or drug users can serve as triggers for women to drink or use drugs.

The choice is yours. Do you want to decide when and how much you drink or use drugs, or do you want other people to decide? Learning to manage triggers related to heavy drinkers and drug users in your social network will help you decide for yourself.

EXERCISE 3.1
Social Support Network

In this exercise, you will help group members think more about their social networks and the influence of others on their own drinking or drug use. For this exercise, you will be using Handout 3.2: Your Social Network Example and Worksheet 3.2: Your Social Network.

> *The first thing we are going to do today is take a look at your social network to identify who are heavy drinkers or drug users, and how they impact your alcohol/drug use. Then, we will use "self-management planning" sheets so that we can figure out how to cope with that set of interpersonal (i.e., people) triggers.*

Assessing the Social Network

Work out loud with one volunteer group member to start to construct her social network circles:

> *See Handout 3.2: Your Social Network Example and Worksheet 3.2: Your Social Network to make a picture of your social network as you experience it. You see there are circles within circles, with a spot for your name in the middle. Let's see if we can construct a social network for one person here, so that you all can see how it's done. While we're doing an example, you can follow along and fill in your own circle. Would anyone like to volunteer?* [Demonstrate on flipchart.]

> *Write your name in the innermost circle. Write the first names of the person/people you consider closest to you in the closest inner circles, and then move out from there in terms of placement. So, _____, who would you put in the circle closest to you?*

> *The people in the outermost circles would be less close to you than those in the inner circles. Who might go in this next circle? And the next?*

> *This is a picture of your social network.* [Also ask the group: *Is everyone able to fill out theirs?]*

Now, we'll draw a box around those who drink or use drugs at all. Then, we put D, for Heavy Drinker, next to the names of people who you think are currently heavy drinkers, and we put DRU, for Drug User or drug problem, next to the names of people who use drugs. _____, who in your network is a heavy drinker? A drug user? As we are labeling _____'s circle, follow along on your own worksheet, using your own social network. Put ALC (for alcohol problem) next to the names of people you think have an alcohol problem. [Also ask the group: *How did everyone else do?*]

When you and the volunteer client have completed the worksheet, elicit discussion about the social network support exercise from both the volunteer and other group members.

HANDOUT 3.2

Your Social Network Example

Sue

Kevin, Brother — DRU / D
Dad — ALC
Mom
Dan, Husband — ALC
Shari, Best Friend — D
Lucy, Cousin — D
Joey & Shelley, Friends — D
Karen, Sis-In-Law — ALC
Lois, Friend
Drew, Cousin
Sasha, Co-Worker

D = Heavy Drinker
DRU = Drug User or Drug Problem
ALC = Alcohol Problem

WORKSHEET 3.2
Your Social Network

D = Heavy Drinker
DRU = Drug User or Drug Problem
ALC = Alcohol Problem

Presence of Heavy Drinkers/Drug Users in Social Network

You should make some observations about the volunteer's social network graphic. For example:

> *No wonder you had a tough week of triggers! Looking at this picture, I can see that most of the people in your inner circles are either heavy drinkers or have an alcohol or drug problem. You have a strong set of interpersonal triggers to deal with, and that usually makes it hard to stop drinking/using and stay sober/clean. That's exactly why we did this exercise, to clarify who might be an interpersonal trigger for you, and then we'll figure out how to deal with that.*

Next, take a look around the room at other completed circles, and point out at least one other example that illustrates social network members who don't drink or use drugs, but are further out in the outermost circles, to comment on the possibility that the client might think about how to develop more contact with people who don't use alcohol or drugs.

> *This exercise is also a chance to step back and see a graphic of your social network in general to check if you have enough supportive people in your life, and we will discuss in Session 8 how to make more supportive connections. For instance, if you see someone in your circles who you feel close to and miss, but rarely get to see or talk to them, maybe you might want to brainstorm about how to interact with that person more often (in person, or maybe schedule remote video chat coffee dates or calls, or text more often, for instance).*

▪ **Question:** Can we list other group members in our network?

THERAPIST: *Good question. This exercise is meant to reflect your social network as it is outside of this group, so if you have contact with other group members outside of the group sessions, that's fine. Part of the reason we use a group format to treat women is so you can get some social support here for not drinking or using drugs. So, as you go through this therapy, if you feel you would like to add any group members to your social network, please feel free. We hope that you will serve as supports for each other even after this group ends.*

For homework, ask group members to complete Worksheet 3.3: Heavy Drinkers/Drug Users in Your Social Network.

Therapist Note

If a client says she has no heavy drinkers or drug users in her social network, still have her complete the exercise, and have her add people who may be outside of her intimate social network, but still may be triggers for her. Then, use self-management planning (introduced later in this session) for those.

EXERCISE 3.2
Assessing the Impact of Your Social Network on Change Efforts

In this exercise, you will guide clients through thinking more about the impact of heavy drinkers and drug users on their own use and efforts to change. For this exercise, you will be using Handout 3.3: Heavy Drinkers/Drug Users in Your Social Network: Sample and Worksheet 3.3: Heavy Drinkers/Drug Users in Your Social Network.

> *Now let's look at Handout 3.3 and Worksheet 3.3. I'd like you to think about three or four people who are most important to you, and to think about how they might affect your efforts to change your drinking or drug use. Later on, we'll be working on new ways to interact with them.*

Ask for a volunteer to complete the worksheet out loud for at least one person in her network. Then, ask group members to do the same, sharing what they are writing down.

Name of heavy drinker/drug user ___Shari___

How might this person's drinking affect your efforts to stop drinking/using drugs and stay sober?

We usually get together once a week for dinner or happy hour. She'll be upset if I don't go with her and I don't think she'd understand why I'm not drinking. She's my best friend; we've been partying together since our 20s. I don't think I can go to happy hour with her anymore, and maybe not even restaurants.

Name of heavy drinker/drug user ___Kevin, Karen___

How might this person's drinking affect your efforts to stop drinking/using drugs and stay sober?

My brother and sister-in-law and I always get together before family events to talk about our parents—we need a few drinks to prepare ourselves. Kevin and Karen also smoke weed. They get smashed. I think they'll be offended and pushy if I don't drink with them, and this will be a high-risk situation for me.

Name of heavy drinker/drug user ___Dan___

How might this person's drinking affect your efforts to stop drinking/using drugs and stay sober?

Dan's my biggest problem when it comes to my stopping drinking. He and I drink together almost daily; it's part of our relationship. I know he needs to stop too, but he doesn't see that.

Name of heavy drinker/drug user ___Joey and Shelley___

How might this person's drinking affect your efforts to stop drinking/using drugs and stay sober?

Dan and I see Joey and Shelley twice a month, and everyone drinks a lot. It will be hard to find other activities we all enjoy other than going to a bar.

WORKSHEET 3.3
Heavy Drinkers/ Drug Users in Your Social Network

Name of heavy drinker/drug user _____

    How might this person's drinking affect your efforts to stop drinking/using drugs and stay sober?

_____

_____

_____

_____

Name of heavy drinker/drug user _____

    How might this person's drinking affect your efforts to stop drinking/using drugs and stay sober?

_____

_____

_____

_____

Name of heavy drinker/drug user _____

    How might this person's drinking affect your efforts to stop drinking/using drugs and stay sober?

_____

_____

_____

_____

Name of heavy drinker/drug user _____

    How might this person's drinking affect your efforts to stop drinking/using drugs and stay sober?

_____

_____

_____

_____

Rationale:

Now let's discuss a method I want to teach you called "self-management planning" as a way to cope with drinking or drug use triggers.

Paraphrase:

Self-management planning is a problem-solving technique to help you figure out ways to deal with specific triggers to make life less risky for drinking/drug use.

Self-management planning is aimed at teaching the client to alter triggers to decrease the likelihood that she will drink/use drugs in response to these cues, or to learn new ways to respond to the triggers. This means thinking of ways to rearrange those environmental events that have triggered drinking or drug use in the past, or to replace them with non-risky situations. The antecedents were identified through self-recording, functional analysis, and clients' observations of their own reactions. Self-management planning focuses on settings or situations, times, and people, rather than thoughts and feelings. Naturally, these categories are related to each other, and several can be going on at the same time. For some clients only a subset of these antecedents will applicable. Refer to Handout 3.4: How to Manage Triggers, and group members can follow along as you explain. Jot down important points on the flipchart.

Also emphasize the following:

Self-management is a great skill to use because it enables you to take charge of your situation and be active *and "planful" in coming up with solutions that work for you. You are not a victim of circumstance. Of course, you can't control if certain triggers—most triggers, in fact—just happen. But you* can *control how you respond to those triggers, and you can control* your *actions. We want you to give up feeling bad about triggers you can't control and put your energies into your reactions, which you* can *control!*

HANDOUT 3.4
How to Manage Triggers

We have spent some time talking about triggers. We know they come in all shapes and sizes. Some lead to very strong urges/cravings. Some involve loved ones; others come from our daily routines. Some triggers lead to very difficult situations, but others are easier to handle.

- Knowing about triggers is not enough.
  We need a plan!

- Developing a good plan takes patience and a lot of thinking.
  We have a step-by-step method that makes planning much easier.

- You probably have personal triggers and triggers related to your relationships.

1. **Pick out triggers that you will come across soon.** Start with an easier trigger. As you get more practice at this, you can plan for harder triggers.

2. **Write down as many ideas as possible for handling the trigger.** Be creative! Do not worry about being silly or unrealistic. The best ideas often come when you let ideas fly without stopping to think about what is good or bad about each one. The evaluation will come later. There are three kinds of strategies for handling triggers:

   - **Remove yourself from the situation to avoid trouble.**

   - **Change things around you to avoid the trigger.** For example, get rid of alcohol or drugs around the house or do not walk past the liquor store.

   - **Think or act in different ways when you are faced with the trigger.** For example, someone may avoid drinking or using drugs by remembering the consequences that will come later.

3. *After* **coming up with a lot of ideas, think and write down what is good and bad about each one.** Now is the time to think about what you need to do for each one of the ideas. Remember, some consequences of your plan will happen quickly, and others will happen later. Try to think them through. The goal here is to think about what is good and bad about each idea.

4. **Think about how easy or hard each idea would be for you to implement.** Some ideas will be hard to do, while others will be easy. For each idea or plan, give it a number between 1 and 10 that shows how hard it would be to do. For example, the easiest plan that you can do would get a 1. The hardest thing that you could do would get a 10. Write down how easy or hard each idea would be for you. That is, how difficult would it be to carry out the new plan in place of old behavior that involved drinking or using drugs in response to the trigger?

5. **Pick a plan.** Choose the plan or plans that have the best balance between positive and negative consequences. Try to pick ones that will not be too hard for you.

6. **After putting a plan to work, check to see how it is working.** If a plan is not working, do not be afraid to make changes or to pick another idea.

Now it is your turn. On Worksheet 3.4: Self-Management Planning, put down your top triggers and build your plan. Follow our system as you go through the planning.

EXERCISE 3.3
Self-Management Planning: Description

For this exercise, you and the clients will need Handout 3.5: Self-Management Planning: Example 1, Handout 3.6: Self-Management Planning: Example 2, and Worksheet 3.4: Self-Management Planning.

Review the sample completed self-management plans for heavy drinkers or drug users in the social network using Handouts 3.5 and 3.6. Highlight the procedure used to construct self-management plans:

- For each trigger, decide on the best management strategy: avoidance, rearrangement, new coping method, other.
- Consider the overall effects that the proposed strategy would have on the client's life and lifestyle goals.
- Rate the predicted difficulty of using each strategy or plan (e.g., some plans can be implemented with minimal environmental modifications, while others may require a short-term avoidance strategy followed by long-term learning of alternative responses). Note that the difficulty rating refers to the difficulty of carrying out the new plan instead of the old behavior that involved drinking or drug use in response to the trigger.

HANDOUT 3.5
Self-Management Planning: Example 1

Trigger	Plan	Positive/Negative Consequences	Difficulty* (1–10)
Partner invites neighbors over for impromptu barbecue at our house; they are all pot smokers. My partner asks me to roll a few joints for everyone while I tend the grill.	a. Abandon efforts to stay sober and join them	a. Positive: Have fun, fit in; not embarrassed that I am not smoking Negative: Let myself down; cravings restart; later resentful of partner	a. 4t
	b. Leave home until the party is over	b. Positive: Avoid trigger; avoid smoking Negative: No one sober is watching the kids at home; partner annoyed, neighbors baffled; resentful of partner	b. 8
	c. Make myself a non-alcoholic drink and stay busy at the grill and in the kitchen	c. Positive: Socialize; enjoy a non-alcoholic drink; partner not annoyed Negative: Still a high-risk situation, high cravings; resentment toward partner	c. 5
	d. Approach partner the following week and discuss this and similar situations with her	d. Positive: Express feelings, be assertive; possibly avoid future similar situations; plan ahead Negative: Partner may not wish to talk about it; may be frustrating	d. 10
	e. Remain pleasant to neighbors but don't join the barbecue; stay inside. Tell your partner you won't be rolling any joints.	e. Positive: Avoid trigger; protecting right to self-care Negative: Bored, resentful of partner; partner annoyed	e. 10

* Difficulty of carrying out the plan in this context

HANDOUT 3.6
Self-Management Planning: Example 2

Trigger	Plan	Positive/Negative Consequences	Difficulty* (1–10)
1. Going to restaurant with husband	a. Do not go	a. Positive: Avoid trigger Negative: No fun; husband resentful	a. 9
	b. Go to restaurant that does not serve liquor	b. Positive: Avoid trigger Negative: Husband may not agree; may not like food	b. 3
	c. Learn to refuse when husband or waiter urges you to order a drink	c. Positive: Don't need to switch restaurants Negative: May feel uncomfortable; still faced with difficult trigger	c. 8
2. Keeping liquor in the house	a. Never buy liquor	a. Positive: Save money; avoid trigger Negative: Husband can't drink at home; company can't drink	a. 5
	b. Have spouse hide the liquor	b. Positive: Avoid trigger Negative: Inconvenient; liquor still in house	b. 9
	c. Don't invite people who drink	c. Positive: Avoid trigger Negative: Lose friends	c. 8
	d. Don't serve liquor to guests	d. Positive: Save money; put yourself first Negative: Some may be offended	d. 7
	e. Buy liquor before guests come and throw out the extra right after	e. Positive: Avoid offending guests; minimize exposure to trigger Negative: May waste money	e. 2

* Difficulty of carrying out the plan in this context

Continue the session by asking the group the following questions:

What is your reaction to these self-management plans? Is there anything you would have added? Sometimes women want to please others and are hesitant to assert their needs—see Session 9 if you need help with assertiveness to carry out your plans.

Next you will generate some brief discussion about self-management planning:

Now, let's do a self-management plan together. In our last exercise, we discussed heavy drinkers/drug users in your social network. Does anyone want to volunteer their heavy drinker/drug user situation for this self-management planning exercise? Great, thanks, _____.

Elicit a range of plans and positive and negative consequences from the group. Ask the volunteer to rank the difficulty of each plan.

What is everyone's reaction to this exercise? For homework, complete a self-management plan for at least one trigger using Worksheet 3.4.

WORKSHEET 3.4

Self-Management Planning

Trigger	Plan	Positive/Negative Consequences	Difficulty* (1–10)
1.			
2.			

* Difficulty of carrying out the plan in this context

Farewell to Members Leaving the Group (10 minutes)

Have members who are leaving identify the skills they think have been most important to the changes that they have made during therapy—that is, those skills they will continue to try to implement in order to maintain their progress. Remind group members that relapses most often occur in the types of situations they are now prepared to handle.

For women finishing the group, ask them how they feel about finishing the treatment program. Explore termination issues—fear, relief, loss. Discuss referrals for additional treatment if necessary. Discuss the possibility that group members may wish to stay in contact and provide support to one another.

Each group member who is finishing treatment should also be asked to go around the room and say something positive or constructive to each of her fellow group members. These statements could focus on positive changes or steps the leaving group member has seen each of the other women make during treatment, or ways in which the leaving group member feels she herself has learned or benefited from other women in the group. Other group members also should be encouraged to give some positive feedback to the woman who is finishing treatment. Women who are finishing treatment and the therapist may also want to say something to one another.

Anticipating High-Risk Situations This Week (5 minutes)

Rationale:

At the end of each session, we will spend a bit of time discussing any problem situations that each member thinks might come up around drinking or drug use this week. As you each progress through therapy, you will get better and better at anticipating and handling these. A "high-risk situation" is a situation in which you would find it very difficult not to drink. Today, I'd like us each to spend a few minutes together thinking about the upcoming week. [For each group member:] Are there any situations that you might encounter this week that would tempt you to drink or use drugs?

EXERCISE 3.4
High-Risk Situations and Executing High-Risk Situation Plans

Use Worksheet 3.5: High-Risk Situations, located in the Client Workbook.

Now let's each use Worksheet 3.5: High-Risk Situations to write in a high-risk situation for this upcoming week and brainstorm together about strategies/solutions you can use to cope with that high-risk situation in order to avoid drinking or using drugs in response to it. Are there any situations that you might encounter this week that would tempt you to drink or use drugs?

Elicit examples of upcoming high-risk situations from members and brainstorm together to generate plans for how to handle the situation for two or three group members. Write ideas about how to handle this situation on the High-Risk Situations worksheet. Refer to Session 1 in this guide for a copy of the worksheet or to the Client Workbook (Worksheet 3.5) for a client version of the worksheet.

Assign Homework (5 minutes)

Here is a list of homework assignments for each group member to complete between today's session and the next. Remind the women how important it is to complete the homework.

1. Complete one self-monitoring card each day.
2. On the back of your self-monitoring cards, write down high-risk situations you encountered and how you handled them
3. Complete behavior chains (Worksheet 3.1) for two more "real-life" triggers during the week.
4. Complete Worksheet 3.3: Heavy Drinkers/Drug Users in Your Social Network.
5. Complete Worksheet 3.4 for at least one trigger.
6. Complete Worksheet 3.5: High-Risk Situations, located in the Client Workbook, and execute high-risk situation plans.

CHAPTER 9

Session 4: Enhancing Motivation to Change and Increasing Positive Consequences of Abstinence

(Corresponds to Chapter 4 in the Client Workbook)
(1.5 hours)

Notes to the Therapist Before the Session

1. For rolling-admission groups (see Chapter 3), each new member should have an individual assessment (see Chapter 5) with the group facilitator prior to joining the group. At the end of the assessment session, for women joining the group at any session (i.e., Session 2–12) after Session 1, the therapist should spend an additional 30 minutes with each new group member to provide the Client Workbook and to review basic information covered in Session 1 that the client will need to know to proceed with all subsequent sessions. This includes coverage of use of the Client Workbook and group rules, as well as a brief review of core treatment elements, including self-monitoring, psychoeducation, high-risk situations, triggers, and behavior chains (see Session 2). That way, no matter what session the new member is entering, she will be able to do daily self-monitoring and understand the basics of high-risk situations, triggers, and behavior chains.

2. Each rolling-admission group session with a new member starts with a 5-minute round robin introduction of each group member, and 10 minutes of assessment feedback to the new member(s) (see Session 1 for detailed instructions and feedback sheets). Members in the group at different stages of recovery can provide support to the new client and share their own feedback from their first session. If a new member

is lacking relevant information from previous sessions, she can review sessions in the Client Workbook or you can briefly describe the section, and/or abstinent members can be encouraged to spend time with the new member after session to explain relevant prior material.

3. For each new member entering the group in Sessions 2 to 12, follow instructions at the beginning of each session regarding Introductions and Providing Assessment Feedback in Client's First Session.

4. If this is a client's first session, you must summarize data from the pretreatment assessment to fill in a Feedback Sheet (see Handout 1.10 in Client Workbook) for each client in the group in preparation for her first session.

5. Before the session begins, write the session agenda on a flipchart, whiteboard, or blackboard.

6. If you are doing the Optional Graphing Intervention, see instructions in Chapter 3 of this Therapist Guide.

7. All worksheets and handouts used in this treatment program appear in this Therapist Guide and in the corresponding Client Workbook; worksheets (and selected handouts) can also be accessed by searching for this book's title on the Oxford Academic platform, at academic.oup.com.

Session 4 Outline

All times are approximate and should be adjusted based on clinical need and whether group time needs to be devoted to new or departing members.

1. Pre-session sign-in and substance use check (15 minutes before session begins)

2. Introductions and agenda setting (5 minutes)

3. Check-in, review of self-monitoring and homework (20 minutes)

4. Decisional matrix and rearranging positive consequences of abstinence (50 minutes)

5. Farewell to members leaving the group (10 minutes)

6. Anticipating high-risk situations this week (10 minutes)

7. Assign homework (5 minutes)

1. Flipchart, whiteboard, or blackboard, felt-tip markers or chalk, eraser
2. Breathalyzer and tubes or saliva strips (optional)
3. Saliva drug tests for each group member (optional)
4. Seven self-monitoring cards for each group member (Note to therapist: Keep a stack of these to give group members at each session.)
5. OPTIONAL: Individualized graph for each woman
6. Handouts
   4.1: The Good, the Bad, and the Ugly of Drinking and Drug Use
   4.2: Decisional Matrix: Sample
   4.3: Pleasurable Activities: What Do Other People Do?
7. Worksheets
   4.1: Decisional Matrix
   4.2: My Positive and Negative Consequences Reminder Card
   4.3: Alternatives to Drinking or Using Drugs
   4.4: High-Risk Situations [See Client Workbook Worksheet 4.4]

Pre-Session Sign-In and Substance Use Check (15 minutes pre-session)

If any member of the group appears to be high or intoxicated, you may want to assess her blood alcohol level (BAL) with a breathalyzer or saliva strip or use a saliva drug screen. Regardless of formal testing, though, if a group member is visibly high or intoxicated, review the treatment agreement with her and let her know that she will be not be allowed to attend this session. Clients who miss a session will not receive a make-up session, but encourage them to read the handouts they missed for that session and complete the homework for the following week. You should assist the client in arranging alternate transportation home, review her abstinence plan, and remind her of her abstinence goal.

Introductions and Agenda Setting (5 minutes)

You will introduce new members joining the group this session, and provide an overview (i.e., set agenda) of what will be covered in the session: *Today we will talk about the pros and cons of drinking/using drugs or not, and coming up with other ways to fulfill the function of substances in your life. We will also discuss how to make an abstinent life more pleasant.* Ask group members if there is anything pressing they would like to discuss today in addition to the planned material. Explain the absence of missing members without revealing protected health information.

Check-In, Review of Self-Monitoring and Homework (20 minutes)

Check-in follows a "round robin" format, in which drinking status and homework are emphasized. To introduce the round robin check-in:

We're going to go around the room using what we call a "round robin check-in" to get a brief version of how your week has been, focusing on your alcohol use, drug use, cravings, and triggers; how you coped with triggers and cravings; in hindsight what you might have done differently (with therapist and group input/ideas as well); homework you completed and what was helpful about it. We also will answer or clarify any questions or concerns about the homework material. Each group member will have a few minutes [depending on how many women there are in the group] to discuss with the group how your coping with alcohol/drug use triggers has been this week.

> **Therapist Note**
> *Try to pay particular attention to women's specific themes (e.g., right to self-care, empowerment) to link experiences to the specific theme: "One theme I've heard that's common among several of you is . . ."*

Go around the room and ask each group member how her week was (focusing on alcohol and/or drug use); listen while looking over her self-monitoring cards; and link what she is saying to her daily cards for alcohol/drug cravings, triggers, and use. Use information from this for specific topics in the rest of the session. Check in with each group member and discuss the progress of her abstinence plan. Update the plan if necessary. Also remember to ask each client at the end of her round robin time about what homework she was able to complete.

You should reinforce self-recording behavior, check for questions or problems, and help group members develop solutions for difficulties related to self-recording procedures. Ask members if they have any questions. Possible questions to anticipate include:

- **Question:** I thought about drinking the whole morning. Is that one urge or more than one?

THERAPIST: *You had the urge continually?*

CLIENT: Not every minute.

THERAPIST: *Well, each time you have a thought or an image about having a specific type of drink or a drink in a particular situation, that counts as a separate urge. Can you share some specific situations you thought about?*

- **Question:** Why are my urges so much higher than everyone else's? Why am I the only one still drinking?

THERAPIST: *It's natural that you would want to compare your drinking/ drug use and urges to those of the other group members. Although this can be an important motivator, it also is important to remember that everyone has her own unique path to abstinence. You're working on it, so be patient with yourself, and think of the changes you've already made! What does the group think about what _____ said?*

Therapist Note

After reviewing the daily monitoring cards, for outpatient settings you may wish to include the optional Graphing Intervention here.

Optional Graphing Intervention for Outpatient Treatment Settings

See the detailed instructions in Chapter 3 of this guide for how to use the graphs located in Session 2 of the Therapist Guide and in the Client Workbook (Handout 2.1. Graph: Alcohol/Drug Use and Urges Sample and Worksheet 2.1. Graph: Alcohol/Drug Use and Urges). This intervention will allow each woman to track her progress by entering weekly data summarized from her daily monitoring cards: 1. Number of drinks; 2. Number of drugs used; 3. Number of urges/cravings; and 4. Average strength of urges/cravings.

Other Homework Review

Review all other homework clients did during the prior week. Reinforce clients for completing homework and discuss barriers experienced in completing the homework. Ask questions such as, *"What did you learn from the homework?"* or *"How can you use the homework to help you in the future?"*

Remember that as part of homework review, each week you need to review group members' recording of high-risk situations and how these were handled: *"Who wants to share how you handled one of your high-risk situations this week without drinking/using drugs?"* Elicit high-risk examples from two or three group members and get feedback from other members. Remember to have group members direct their comments to the other group members, and not just to you. Point out common types of high-risk situations among the group members and encourage women facing similar situations to share how they coped or ideas for coping. Selectively model and repeat empowering and motivational positive affirmations that group members give to one another: for example, *"We know this is hard, you're doing great." "Next time you'll be able to use a different strategy, hang in there."*

Also, ask about progress with doctor's appointments and blood tests. Due to time constraints, group members should discuss any concerns about their blood test or feedback with you after the group. Ask each client to bring in a copy of her lab results and give it to you. You can give feedback to the client during review of homework either that week or the week after.

Therapist Note

You should manage participation so that there is enough time to go around the room in a round robin fashion and give each group member a chance to speak. Keep in mind that 10 to 30 minutes total is allotted for check-in depending on how many women are in the group. If homework is not done, you should ask what made it difficult for the client to complete the homework. The importance of completing homework should be discussed, and a firm commitment for the future should be stressed in a nonjudgmental way.

Share the following with the group:

The time in the treatment group is only part of the process. The real change occurs when you practice changing your lives in the real world. The group will help you get ideas, stay motivated, keep you on track, and develop an understanding of the problem. But actually changing behavior takes place in your everyday life—at home, at work, with family, friends, and so on.

Therapist Note

The following are some tips for managing members' participation to maintain the temporal structure of the session: For habitually quiet members or those who appear upset or distressed, you should acknowledge them with empathic nonverbal behavior, but do not call on them to elicit participation right away, except during their turn in the round robin. Look for opportunities to invite limited participation of habitually quiet members to help them become comfortable sharing. Frequently ask the group for their feedback on particular group members' contributions, to set up the expectation that group members will be doing a lot of the work in the room. Everyone in the group learns by hearing the experiences and advice of others. Model and facilitate a tone of supportive, constructive, and compassionate feedback in the group. Don't be confrontational, but also don't condone or reassure a woman about her drinking/drug use or lack of work outside the group sessions. For instance, don't say, "It's okay. You had a really hard week; of course you drank a bit." Say instead, "You certainly had a hard week! In hindsight, what could you have done differently in response to trigger xxx?"

Group members who are having substantial difficulty with their abstinence plan or who appear to be at risk for an emergency should be asked discreetly to remain after group for an individual check-in with you.

Decisional Matrix and Rearranging Positive Consequences of Abstinence (50 minutes)

Rationale: The goal of this exercise is to enhance the group members' motivation to make or maintain changes in their alcohol or drug use, to increase their focus on reasons to change ("change talk"), and to decrease their focus on reasons not to change ("sustain talk"). This treatment is not formal motivational interviewing (MI), but you should incorporate certain aspects of MI into the discussion (see also Chapter 4). You can draw on several elements of "MI spirit," which we routinely use as we work collaboratively with each client in high-quality cognitive behavioral therapy (CBT). These collaborative elements include creating a partnership between you and the group members; accepting each group member's inherent worth as a person, expressed through empathy and support for their ability to change; communicating your compassion for the challenges they face; and placing an emphasis on evoking their own reasons to change. Several specific therapeutic techniques may help you in using a collaborative CBT approach and "MI spirit":

(1) Asking open-ended rather than close-ended questions will draw the women out. Open-ended rather than yes/no questions encourage a person to talk—for example, "How does your family fit into your reasons to change?" versus "Is your family one of your reasons to change?"

(2) Reflective listening also will help to draw group members out. Reflections may be simple restatements of what a group member has said, with a tone of compassion (e.g., "Your family is an important reason for you to want to change"). At times, you also may use "complex reflections" in which you reflect something that you inferred from what the group member said (e.g., "Your family is an important reason for you to want to change, and you hope it's not too late").

(3) Be on the lookout for change talk and selectively reinforce it through reflective listening and helping group members elaborate more on their reasons to change. Change talk comes in many

forms, including *desire* (e.g., "I want to stop using drugs once and for all"), *ability* (e.g., "I know how to stop—I've done it before"), *reasons* (e.g., "I want my children to respect me"), *need* (e.g., "I'm not getting any younger and I'm worried that, if I keep drinking the way I have been, I'm going to get sick"), and *commitment* (e.g., "I told my daughter I'm coming to this group and we're going to go out to lunch tomorrow so I can share what I'm learning here").

(4) Be careful not to reinforce sustain talk, and avoid letting the group get into extended discussions of reasons not to change. Sustain talk comes in forms similar to change talk, but it is all about maintaining alcohol or drug use rather than changing. Most clients experience some ambivalence about change, and when they express reasons not to change, you can selectively focus on reasons for change that they have expressed while also acknowledging their ambivalence (e.g., "You're worried that you won't be able to sleep without alcohol, *and* you've decided that you need to make a change even if you don't sleep well for a while because alcohol is causing so many problems in your life").

Keep these elements of a collaborative, motivation-enhancing approach in mind as you have clients follow along with Handout 4.1: The Good, the Bad, and the Ugly of Drinking and Drug Use.

Say to the group:

> Even though you have entered treatment, you probably have some mixed feelings about being here and about actually making major changes in your life. This is a common feeling—you don't know what things will be like in the future, and that makes it somewhat frightening. In contrast, you **do** know what things are like now. Sometimes the familiar is comforting, even if it is unhappy. You also are giving up something that has provided enjoyable things in your life: Most people get some pleasure from their drinking or drug use—they enjoy the taste, like the sensations, or associate it with many good things in their lives. Giving it up is like saying goodbye to a friend you will miss, even though we all

know that alcohol and drugs are not friends who have our best interests in mind. Although having mixed feelings about giving up alcohol or drugs is perfectly natural, these feelings don't mean you should keep using alcohol or drugs.

You also may have mixed feelings about abstinence. Some people feel that it's impossible to have fun without alcohol or drugs, or feel that it's the only way they can relax.

I'd like to help you each think out some of the pros and cons of stopping your drinking/drug use and of continuing your drinking/drug use. In thinking about the pros and cons, it may be helpful to think about short-term consequences and longer-term consequences. [Refer to Handout 4.1.]

Therapist Note

Some contemporary motivational interviewing strategies no longer include the decisional matrix. We believe, however, that the decisional matrix is an important intervention to help clients: (1) identify and acknowledge the function of alcohol/drugs in their lives so that they can then find other ways to fulfill those same functions; (2) identify and acknowledge the loss they feel in giving up alcohol or drugs to process/grieve that loss and learn to replace the loss with more positive ways to use their time and energies; (3) consolidate reasons to stop drinking/using drugs and to remain abstinent; and (4) become more acutely aware of the positive consequences of not drinking/using drugs, since this is a crucial motivator to prevent relapse.

HANDOUT 4.1
The Good, the Bad, and the Ugly of Drinking and Drug Use

Why do you want to quit drinking or drug use?

Before we go on, look at the good and bad things about your drinking or drug use. You probably have mixed feelings about stopping drinking or using drugs. It will help you stay motivated if you know why you want to quit.

- **Think about what will be good and bad in the future about quitting drinking or drugs now.** You will be more successful if you look ahead to see the future impact of making a change now. This allows you to process the loss that giving up alcohol/drugs may entail, and also helps you see how advantages of abstinence outweigh the losses.
- **Think about the consequences of your drinking or drug use.** You learned from doing behavior chains that most of the time the good consequences happen right as you drink or use, and the bad consequences come later.
- **There are reasons why you drink/use drugs.** These come from the good things that happen, even if the good things only happen sometimes. Your mind and body remember these things.
- **The bad consequences can come right when you are drinking or using** (like getting sick or having a fight) **or can come later** (like not being able to get up the next morning or having your children upset with you).
- **It will be easier to quit if you have a list of the positives that come with abstinence, and also of the negative aspects of drinking or drug use.** The more you remember the positives of stopping and the bad things that can happen with continued use, the easier it is to say "no" when you have an urge/craving to drink or use.

Some examples of positives of stopping might be: waking up in morning with no hangover; feeling more clear-headed; able to be present emotionally for my kids; saving money; relationship more positive with my spouse; feel better about myself, etc.

Some negative consequences of continuing to drink or use drugs might be related to:

√ Physical things: body sensations or effects like getting sick	√ Things that happen with other people, such as family or friends
√ Emotional feelings	√ Money or legal trouble
√ Depressing thoughts	√ Work problems

Look at Handout 4.2 to see a sample completed decisional matrix. Then, use Worksheet 4.1: Decisional Matrix to write down the good and bad things that will happen in *the short term* when you stop drinking/using drugs. Then write down the good and bad things *that may happen later*, in the longer term. Write these in the section marked *Abstinence*.

Then do the same thing for continuing to drink or use drugs: Write down the good and bad things that happen *right away* (immediate consequences) when you drink or use. Also write down the good and bad things that happen later (delayed consequences; i.e., in the long term) after drinking or using. Write these in the section marked *Continued Alcohol or Drug Use*.

Be realistic! It is important to be honest and also to be specific. The more we understand the reasons why you drink or use drugs, the easier it will be to find solutions.

Abstinence

Pros (short- and long-term)	Cons (short- and long-term)
The only way to end cravings for good in the long run is to not drink or use drugs	Will have to struggle with cravings to use
Won't dial drunk and feel ashamed and embarrassed the next day	Will have to face feeling depressed and anxious without immediate escape
My kids will be proud of me.	
Feel less anxious not doing illegal things (cocaine)	
Will breathe better without weed and cigarettes	
When I drink I want to smoke weed, smoke cigs, and do cocaine. so I'll be less likely to use other drugs	
I'll be there for my kids, more present.	
I can't resolve my trauma damage until I stop self-medicating with alcohol.	
Will be more clear-headed and feel better, especially in the mornings	
Able to act in accord 2=with my values and who I want to be	

Continued Alcohol or Drug Use

Pros (short- and long-term)	Cons (short- and long-term)
To piss off Mateo when I'm angry at him	Alcohol and cocaine expensive
Don't have to struggle with cravings to use	Cocaine dangerous—heart attack risk
Avoid withdrawal symptoms in short term	Drinking actually keeps cravings alive.
Tastes good	Weight gain—eat more when drunk or high
Immediate relaxation and escape from depression/anxiety	Feel terrible most mornings—hung over, headache, foggy
I like the feeling of being high, or used to.	Ashamed of myself in front of Mateo and the kids and my parents
	I am not being who I want to be.
	Hate feeling out of control of my use
	I almost never even feel high anymore. It's not worth it.

EXERCISE 4.1
Decisional Matrix

In this exercise, you will help group members think through the pros and cons of changing their use of alcohol/drugs, and the pros and cons of continuing to use. A goal of this exercise is to reinforce clients' commitment to change. For this exercise, you will be using Handout 4.2: Decisional Matrix: Sample and Worksheet 4.1: Decisional Matrix.

Ask group members whether or not they can relate to the sample comments in Handout 4.2, and encourage discussion. After some general discussion, ask for a volunteer to go over the pros and cons of abstinence and of continued drinking/drug use with you using the flipchart/whiteboard/blackboard. Before having group members follow along and jot down their own pros and cons on their worksheet, have them take out Worksheet 4.2, and explain it to the group. Then, work with the volunteer, using the flipchart, and have her and the other group members identify some good and bad things about abstinence and then also about continuing to use alcohol or drugs. By this time in therapy, you should be well acquainted with the client's drinking or drug use pattern and the function of alcohol/drugs in her life, so you can help her identify pros and cons that are highly personalized and individualized to her personal situation. Group members should be encouraged to chime in and offer suggested pros and cons that might make sense for the volunteer. Instruct group members to also write their own pros and cons on their decisional matrix worksheet as they follow along.

> **Therapist Note**
>
> *In addition to the long-term pros of abstinence the group generates, encourage them to consider these advantages of abstinence:*

- *Feeling more confident, more in control, and better about oneself*
- *Having more time for oneself*
- *Treating oneself and one's body in a healthier way*
- *Feeling more in control of oneself*

> *Also, point out some subtle short-term pros of (reasons for) drinking/using drugs that some women might not be recognizing as motivators to continue using and that you can address in therapy:*

- *Feeling "young again" ("partying")*
- *Filling empty time due to retirement or empty nest*
- *Takes the edge off PMS irritability or menopause mood swings*
- *A way to annoy a loved one with whom you are angry*

Check in again to ask group members if they have questions at this point and to discuss how it was to work on the decisional matrix, before assigning it for homework.

For homework, ask group members to spend more time and complete their decisional matrix worksheet.

WORKSHEET 4.1
Decisional Matrix

Abstinence

Pros (short- and long-term)	Cons (short- and long-term)

Continued Alcohol or Drug Use

Pros (short- and long-term)	Cons (short- and long-term)

Now that we have identified some of the pros and cons of stopping versus continuing to drink or use drugs, let's talk about two ways you can use this decisional matrix to help you become or stay sober.

EXERCISE 4.2

Creating a Personal Card Listing Positive Consequences of NOT Drinking/Using Drugs and Negative Consequences of Drinking/Using Drugs

In this exercise, you will help each client to create a handy summary of her decisional matrix. Your goal is to help group members create something that they can carry around with them to help them keep their most important reasons for change clearly in mind. For this exercise, you will be using Worksheet 4.2: My Positive and Negative Consequences Reminder Card.

Therapist Note
Refer group members to Worksheet 4.2 for the next exercise.

Research suggests that focusing on the positive consequences of NOT using alcohol or drugs helps to keep people from relapsing, so it is very important to identify and remind yourself daily of the benefits you experience from not drinking or using drugs.

*This exercise will help you develop a **habit of thinking** about the **positives of not using** the substance, and also the **cons of drinking or using the drug.** This is one way of managing your thoughts to help you avoid drinking or drug use.*

Pulling from clients' completed decisional matrix worksheets, ask each group member to list positive consequences of NOT drinking/using drugs and negative consequences of drinking or drug use on Worksheet 4.2, and then discuss ways to increase the amount of time each client thinks about these consequences to help her learn a new thinking habit. Suggest that clients read the 3×5 card on Worksheet 4.2 prior to engaging in high-frequency activities (e.g., hang the card on the mirror in the bathroom, put it near the coffeepot or in the car, or add the information into their smartphone as a reminder).

Ask group members to share their ideas about where they will put the card to use it most helpfully. For example:

A friend calls and invites you to join her and a few other people at a bar or restaurant to relax and socialize. Your first thoughts will most probably be related to the positive consequences of drinking (don't be surprised: you've had a long time to develop that thinking habit!). Delay accepting her offer ("I need to check my schedule; let me get back to you in an hour") and review your 3 × 5 card (or list on your phone). Practice your new thinking habit. Then call her back and decline, using these suggestions:

- *Be firm but polite: Make it clear that you mean what you say when you decline.*
- *Suggest an alternative: Even though you aren't going to go to the bar/restaurant, say you'd like to see her and ask if she'd like to go along on your shopping trip on Saturday.*

We look at how to refuse alcohol and drugs and drinking or drug use opportunities in depth in Session 9.

My Positive and Negative Consequences Reminder Card

List the positive consequences of abstinence from alcohol and drugs, and the negative consequences of drinking/drug use on this card. Keep it where you will see it in the course of your day.

Positive Consequences of Abstinence

_____
_____
_____
_____

Negative Consequences of Drinking/Using Drugs

_____
_____
_____
_____
_____
_____

Where I will keep this card: _____

EXERCISE 4.3
Plan Rewarding Alternatives: New Pathways to Getting
Old Positives You Got from Drinking or Drug Use

In this exercise, you will introduce the idea of finding alternative ways to obtain some of the positive consequences that group members used to associate with drinking or drug use. For this exercise, you will be using Handout 4.3: Pleasurable Activities: What Do Other People Do? and Worksheet 4.3: Alternatives to Drinking or Using Drugs.

> *When people develop a drinking or drug problem, they experience a "funneling effect": Many resources—time, money, energy, attention—are directed toward the alcohol or drug use, including thinking about alcohol or drugs, getting alcohol or drugs, using alcohol or drugs, being drunk or high, and recovering from the effects. Women tend to develop this funneling effect fairly quickly after the onset of regular (patterned) drinking or drug use.*

> *When women leave alcohol or drugs behind, they often experience a frightening emptiness in their lives: The time and energy that alcohol or drug use took have to be filled with something rewarding to keep you from going back to drinking or using drugs. Try to think of it like this: One advantage of not drinking or using is that you have newfound freedom to use your time and resources in new ways, in whatever ways you choose. Let's make that a conscious choice. To help you with that, we've listed some activities many people enjoy. Let's take a look at Handout 4.3: Pleasurable Activities: What Do Other People Do? and then take a few minutes to check which activities seem appealing to you to try and/or list some of your own ideas.*

Generate discussion while group members look over Handout 4.3 and discuss what they might like to try during newly free time that used to be taken up by drinking, being intoxicated, or being hung over. Help the group develop a list of options that can serve as positive, rewarding alternatives to drinking or drug use (e.g., relaxation, social activities, enjoying nature). Remind the group that they might select activities that fit with their longer-term goals (for example, one member might decide to go running or do another form of exercise to relax instead of reading or listening to music, if she wants to get into better shape) and goals of self-care.

Pleasurable Activities: What Do Other People Do?

Circle ones you think you might like to do, and add your own at the bottom.

Read a novel	Have a meal with a family member or friend	Practice on a musical instrument or take lessons
Volunteer at an animal shelter	Look at old photos, start a scrapbook	Play cards or board games or video games
Go hiking or take a walk or jog	Try a new recipe, make a nice dinner or bake	Join a social group at a place of worship
Have a picnic	Pray or meditate (try an app)	Sing or listen to music, dance
Spend time by a pool or beach, swim if you like	Plant flowers or a vegetable garden or do yard work	Listen to a podcast
Join or organize a book club	Watch a movie at home, order takeout	Plan a trip to someplace new
Hang out with people you love	Set up a "video chat date" with family members or friends	Bowl, play golf, or bike
Watch TV	Take a walk	Go to a free lecture
Get a manicure, pedicure, or massage	Take your dog to the park	Shopping or browse stores
Go to a sporting event or watch it on TV	Follow an online dance tutorial	Do artwork or a crafting project
Take a nap	See a concert or play	See a movie or show
Sign up for a cooking class or art course	Visit the zoo or aquarium	Go to a museum or art gallery
Take a dance or martial arts or yoga class	Take a drumming class	Browse garage sales or antique shops
Go skating or rollerblading	Join a traditional or online talking circle	Go horseback riding, skiing or snowboarding

Also, let's use the decisional matrix to help you learn to replace the positive things that alcohol or drugs used to do for you. Refer to the list on Worksheet 4.1 (decisional matrix) of the pros of drinking/drug use. We'll think of ways to replace some of the positive consequences of alcohol or drug use with rewarding activities that will be fun, positive, and healthy.

Using Worksheet 4.3: Alternatives to Drinking or Using Drugs, ask for a volunteer to complete a few rows of the worksheet with you, while you use the flip chart to write down what the volunteer is saying. Have the group members suggest alternatives that could provide positive consequences that are similar to the ones the volunteer listed on her decisional matrix. The group members should also follow along on their own worksheet and write down their own alternatives. Discuss with the group the notion that some of the positive consequences of alcohol or drug use, such as euphoria and relaxation induced by alcohol or drugs, are not easily replaced, but that these consequences were artificial and temporary, followed by the negative consequences.

After the volunteer has completed her worksheet, open the discussion up for other group members to share some of the ideas they came up with as their own alternatives that could provide the positive consequences they obtained from drinking or drug use. Let the group members give feedback to one another about their ideas.

WORKSHEET 4.3
Alternatives to Drinking or Using Drugs

Trigger situation and positive consequences of alcohol or drug use: Examples	Alternative activity with similar positive consequence: Examples
a. Saturday night at restaurant with my partner (positive consequences of alcohol: relaxation, wine goes with dinner, euphoria, festive)	a. Make nice dinner at home with partner, then watch a movie at home
b. Tuesday night, my partner working late and no one is home (positive consequence of drug: reduce loneliness, special time alone, relaxation)	b. Go to the gym, then stop on way home at favorite coffee shop for decaf tea.
c. Dinnertime, home cooking (positive consequences of alcohol: habit, makes cooking more fun and festive, feels less boring)	c. Drink my favorite non-alcoholic beverage (cranberry juice with lemon and seltzer) while cooking; put on music while cooking; get takeout or have leftovers 2-3 nights a week and relax with the kids instead of cooking.
d.	d.
e.	e.
f.	f.
g.	g.
h.	h.
i.	i.

Farewell to Members Leaving the Group (10 minutes)

Have members who are leaving identify the skills they think have been most important to the changes that they have made during therapy—that is, those skills they will continue to try to implement in order to maintain their progress. Remind group members that relapses most often occur in the types of situations they are now prepared to handle.

For women finishing the group, ask them how they feel about finishing the treatment program. Explore termination issues—fear, relief, loss. Discuss referrals for additional treatment if necessary. Discuss the possibility that group members may wish to stay in contact and provide support to one another.

Each group member who is finishing treatment should also be asked to go around the room and say something positive or constructive to each of her fellow group members. These statements could focus on positive changes or steps the leaving group member has seen each of the other women make during treatment, or ways in which the leaving group member feels she herself has learned or benefited from other women in the group. Other group members also should be encouraged to give some positive feedback to the woman who is finishing treatment. Women who are finishing treatment and the therapist may also want to say something to one another.

Anticipating High-Risk Situations This Week (10 minutes)

Rationale:

At the end of each session, we will spend a bit of time discussing any problem situations that each member thinks might come up around drinking or drug use this week. As you each progress through therapy, you will get better and better at anticipating and handling these. A "high-risk situation" is a situation in which you would find it very difficult not to drink. Today, I'd like us each to spend a few minutes together thinking about the upcoming week. [For each group member:] Are there any situations that you might encounter this week that would tempt you to drink or use drugs

EXERCISE 4.4
High-Risk Situations and Executing High-Risk Situation Plans

Use Worksheet 4.4: High-Risk Situations, located in the Client Workbook:

Now let's each use Worksheet 4.4: High-Risk Situations to write in a high-risk situation for this upcoming week and brainstorm together about strategies/solutions you can use to cope with that high-risk situation in order to avoid drinking or using drugs in response to it. Are there any situations that you might encounter this week that would tempt you to drink or use drugs?

Elicit examples of upcoming high-risk situations from members and brainstorm together to generate plans for how to handle the situation for two or three group members. Write ideas about how to handle this situation on the High-Risk Situations worksheet. Refer to Session 1 in this guide for a copy of the worksheet or to the Client Workbook (Worksheet 4.4) for a client version of the worksheet.

Assign Homework (5 minutes)

Here is a list of homework assignments for each group member to complete between today's session and the next. Remind the women how important it is to complete the homework.

1. Complete one self-monitoring card each day.
2. On the back of your self-monitoring cards, write down high-risk situations you encountered and how you handled them.
3. Read all the Session 4 material in your workbook and complete worksheets you didn't finish during the session.
4. Review the 3×5 card on Worksheet 4.2: My Positive and Negative Consequences Reminder Card daily.
5. Practice two alternatives to drinking/drug use you had put on Worksheet 4.3: Alternatives to Drinking or Using Drugs.
6. Complete Worksheet 4.4: High-Risk Situations, and execute high-risk situation plans.

CHAPTER 10

Session 5: Well-Being and Self-Care

(Corresponds to Chapter 5 in the Client Workbook)
(1.5 hours)

Notes to the Therapist Before the Session

1. For rolling-admission groups (see Chapter 3), each new member should have an individual assessment (see Chapter 5) with the group facilitator prior to joining the group. At the end of the assessment session, for women joining the group at any session (i.e., Session 2–12) after Session 1, the therapist should spend an additional 30 minutes with each new group member to provide the Client Workbook and to review basic information covered in Session 1 that the client will need to know to proceed with all subsequent sessions. This includes coverage of use of the Client Workbook and group rules, as well as a brief review of core treatment elements, including self-monitoring, psychoeducation, high-risk situations, triggers, and behavior chains (see Session 2). That way, no matter what session the new member is entering, she will be able to do daily self-monitoring and understand the basics of high-risk situations, triggers, and behavior chains.

2. Each rolling-admission group session with a new member starts with a 5-minute round robin introduction of each group member, and 10 minutes of assessment feedback to the new member(s) (see Session 1 for detailed instructions and feedback sheets). Members in the group at different stages of recovery can provide support to the new client and share their own feedback from their first session. If a new member is lacking relevant information from previous sessions, she can review sessions in the Client Workbook or you can briefly

describe the section, and/or abstinent members can be encouraged to spend time with the new member after session to explain relevant prior material.

3. For each new member entering the group in Sessions 2 to 12, follow instructions at the beginning of each session regarding Introductions and Providing Assessment Feedback in Client's First Session.

4. If this is a client's first session, you must summarize data from the pretreatment assessment to fill in a Feedback Sheet (see Handout 1.10 in Client Workbook) for each client in the group in preparation for her first session.

5. Before the session begins, write the session agenda on a flipchart, whiteboard, or blackboard.

6. If you are doing the Optional Graphing Intervention, see instructions in Chapter 3 of this Therapist Guide.

7. All worksheets and handouts used in this treatment program appear in this Therapist Guide and in the corresponding Client Workbook; worksheets (and selected handouts) can also be accessed by searching for this book's title on the Oxford Academic platform, at academic.oup.com.

Session 5 Outline

All times are approximate and should be adjusted based on clinical need and whether group time needs to be devoted to new or departing members.

1. Pre-session sign-in and substance use check (15 minutes before session begins)

2. Introductions and agenda setting (5 minutes)

3. Check-in, review of self-monitoring and homework (10 minutes)

4. Well-being and self-care (65 minutes)

5. Farewell to members leaving the group (10 minutes)

6. Anticipating high-risk situations this week (5 minutes)

7. Assign homework (5 minutes)

1. Flipchart, whiteboard, or blackboard, felt-tip markers or chalk, eraser
2. Breathalyzer and tubes or saliva strips (optional)
3. Saliva drug tests for each group member (optional)
4. Seven self-monitoring cards for each group member (Note to therapist: Keep a stack of these to give group members at each session.)
5. OPTIONAL: Individualized graph for each woman
6. Handouts
   5.1: What Is Self-Care?
   5.2: Self-Compassion Versus Shame
   5.3: Self-Care in My Thoughts: Self-Compassion Versus Shame Automatic Thoughts—Sample
   5.4: Self-Care in My Habits for Well-Being: Behaviors—Sample
   5.5: Lifestyle Want/Should Balance Worksheet—Sample
7. Worksheets
   5.1: Self-Care in My Thoughts: Self-Compassion Versus Shame Automatic Thoughts
   5.2: Self-Care in My Habits for Well-Being: Behaviors
   5.3: Lifestyle Want/Should Balance Worksheet
   5.4: High-Risk Situations [See Client Worksheet 5.4]

Pre-Session Sign-In and Substance Use Check (15 minutes pre-session)

If any member of the group appears to be high or intoxicated, you may want to assess her blood alcohol level (BAL) with a breathalyzer or saliva strip or use a saliva drug screen. Regardless of formal testing, though, if a group member is visibly high or intoxicated, review the treatment agreement with her and let her know that she will not be allowed to attend this session. Clients who miss a session will not receive a make-up session, but encourage them to read the handouts they missed for that session and complete the homework for the following week. You should assist the client in arranging alternate transportation home, review her abstinence plan, and remind her of her abstinence goal.

Introductions and Agenda Setting (5 minutes)

You will introduce new members joining the group this session, and provide an overview (i.e., set agenda) of what will be covered in the session and that the purpose of Session 5 is to discuss well-being, self-care in client thinking, and client behavior. Ask the group if they have anything additional to discuss today.

Check-In, Review of Self-Monitoring and Homework (10 minutes)

Check-in follows a "round robin" format, in which drinking status and homework are emphasized. To introduce the round robin check-in:

We're going to go around the room using what we call a "round robin check-in" to get a brief version of how your week has been, focusing on your alcohol use, drug use, cravings, and triggers; how you coped with triggers and cravings; in hindsight what you might have done differently (with therapist and group input/ideas as well); homework you completed and what was helpful about it. We also will answer or clarify any questions or concerns about the homework material. Each group member will have a few minutes [depending on how many women there are in the group] *to discuss with the group how your coping with alcohol/drug use triggers has been this week.*

Therapist Note

Try to pay particular attention to women's specific themes (e.g., right to self-care, empowerment) to link experiences to the specific theme: "One theme I've heard that's common among several of you is . . ."

Go around the room and ask each group member how her week was (focusing on alcohol and/or drug use); listen while looking over her self-monitoring cards; and link what she is saying to her daily cards for alcohol/drug cravings, triggers, and use. Use information from this for specific topics in the rest of the session. Check in with each group member and discuss the progress of her abstinence plan. Update the plan if necessary. Also remember to ask each client at the end of her round robin time about what homework she was able to complete.

You should reinforce self-recording behavior, check for questions or problems, and help group members develop solutions for difficulties related to self-recording procedures. Ask members if they have any questions. Possible questions to anticipate include:

- **Question:** I thought about drinking the whole morning. Is that one urge or more than one?

THERAPIST: *You had the urge continually?*

CLIENT: Not every minute.

THERAPIST: *Well, each time you have a thought or an image about having a specific type of drink or a drink in a particular situation, that counts as a separate urge. Can you share some specific situations you thought about?*

- **Question:** Why are my urges so much higher than everyone else's? Why am I the only one still drinking?

THERAPIST: *It's natural that you would want to compare your drinking/ drug use and urges to those of the other group members. Although this can be an important motivator, it also is important to remember that everyone has her own unique path to abstinence. You're working on it, so be patient with yourself, and think of the changes you've already made! What does the group think about what _____ said?*

Therapist Note

After reviewing the daily monitoring cards, for outpatient settings you may wish to include the optional Graphing Intervention here.

Optional Graphing Intervention for Outpatient Treatment Settings

See the detailed instructions in Chapter 3 of this guide for how to use the graphs located in Session 2 of the Therapist Guide and in the Client Workbook (Handout 2.1. Graph: Alcohol/Drug Use and Urges Sample [Client Workbook] and Worksheet 2.1. Graph: Alcohol/Drug Use and Urges). This intervention will allow each woman to track her progress by entering weekly data summarized from her daily monitoring cards: 1. Number of drinks; 2. Number of drugs used; 3. Number of urges/cravings; and 4. Average strength of urges/cravings.

Other Homework Review

Review all other homework clients did during the prior week. Reinforce clients for completing homework and discuss barriers experienced in completing the homework. Ask questions such as, *"What did you learn from the homework?"* or *"How can you use the homework to help you in the future?"*

Remember that as part of homework review, each week you need to review group members' recording of high-risk situations and how these were handled: *"Who wants to share how you handled one of your high-risk situations this week without drinking/using drugs?"* Elicit high-risk examples from two or three group members and get feedback from other members. Remember to have group members direct their comments to the other group members, and not just to you. Point out common types of high-risk situations among the group members and encourage women facing similar situations to share how they coped or ideas for coping. Selectively model and repeat empowering and motivational positive affirmations that group members give to one another: for example, *"We know this is hard, you're doing great." "Next time you'll be able to use a different strategy, hang in there."*

Also, ask about progress with doctor's appointments and blood tests. Due to time constraints, group members should discuss any concerns about their blood test or feedback with you after the group. Ask each client to bring in a copy of her lab results and give it to you. You can give feedback to the client during review of homework either that week or the week after.

Therapist Note

You should manage participation so that there is enough time to go around the room in a round robin fashion and give each group member a chance to speak. Keep in mind that 10 to 30 minutes total is allotted for check-in depending on how many women are in the group. If homework is not done, you should ask what made it difficult for the client to complete the homework. The importance of completing homework should be discussed, and a firm commitment for the future should be stressed in a nonjudgmental way.

Share the following with the group:

The time in the treatment group is only part of the process. The real change occurs when you practice changing your lives in the real world. The group will help you get ideas, stay motivated, keep you on track, and develop an understanding of the problem. But actually changing behavior takes place in your everyday life—at home, at work, with family, friends, and so on.

Therapist Note

The following are some tips for managing members' participation to maintain the temporal structure of the session: For habitually quiet members or those who appear upset or distressed, you should acknowledge them with empathic nonverbal behavior, but do not call on them to elicit participation right away, except during their turn in the round robin. Look for opportunities to invite limited participation of habitually quiet members to help them become comfortable sharing. Frequently ask the group for their feedback on particular group members' contributions, to set up the expectation that group members will be doing a lot of the work in the room. Everyone in the group learns by hearing the experiences and advice of others. Model and facilitate a tone of supportive, constructive, and compassionate feedback in the group. Don't be confrontational, but also don't condone or reassure a woman about her drinking/drug use or lack of work outside the group sessions. For instance, don't say, "It's okay. You had a really hard week; of course you drank a bit." Say instead, "You certainly had a hard week! In hindsight, what could you have done differently in response to trigger xxx?"

Group members who are having substantial difficulty with their abstinence plan or who appear to be at risk for an emergency should be asked discreetly to remain after group for an individual check-in with you.

Introduce this material as follows (5 minutes):

Alcohol and drug use takes time, energy, and financial resources; it also creates depression, apathy, anxiety, and isolation. Abstinence from alcohol and drugs is the first step; it's a huge step to clear the path for new ways to use the time, develop new habits, and find new ways to joy and satisfaction.

Having greater psychological well-being is as important as having less stress in your life after alcohol and drugs. It's not just about stopping drinking/drug use and reducing negative moods like depression, irritability, worry, and anxiety. It's also about actively cultivating your ability to feel satisfaction and joy, purpose, meaning, and enjoyment in your life. The way to achieve well-being is through self-care. Learning new thinking habits to "speak to ourselves" with more self-compassion is a form of self-care.

Physical wellness, which is the pursuit of lifestyle habits to achieve good health and quality of life, also is important to well-being. When stopping alcohol and drugs, it helps to swap substance-related unhealthy habits with others such as exercise, mindful nutrition, and other self-care habits. We will help you learn to integrate or increase healthy habits to enhance your physical wellness, which will in turn enhance well-being. We also know that focusing only on the "shoulds" of life without also incorporating pleasant, relaxing, and fun activities robs us of joy in life and results in burnout—fatigue, depression, numbness, and isolation. Self-care is a great method you can use to attain goals of psychological well-being and physical wellness. [Elicit group discussion. Ask questions like: How might the concept of well-being relate to you?]

In this section we will:

- *Learn and practice self-compassionate thinking to facilitate joy and gratitude, and learn to counteract self-criticism (shaming, sometimes even abusive thoughts about ourselves)*
- *Create a list of self-care activities and schedule them into our weekly planners*
- *Complete a "want/should" exercise to help us create a game plan to enjoy a balanced daily lifestyle.*

> **Therapist Note**
>
> *You will be teaching the group this notion: Self-care includes two primary components:*
>
> 1. *Psychological components in our thoughts (e.g., self-compassion vs. shame)*
> 2. *Behavioral components—in our habits*
>   a. *Habits for physical health/wellness include nutrition; exercise; and avoidance of tobacco, alcohol, drugs.*
>   b. *Behavioral habits for well-being/psychological health include pleasant activities, making time for oneself, spending time with a supportive social network, reducing stress, and lifestyle balance (want/should).*
>
> *Let's go through Handout 5.1: What Is Self-Care? together to learn about the two categories of self-care and think about what aspects of self-care you want to continue or start to incorporate into your daily lives.* **Warning:** *You may have to give yourself permission to take care of yourself—it may not come naturally.*

HANDOUT 5.1
What Is Self-Care?

Self-care happens in our thoughts and in our actions (behavior):

- In our thoughts, self-care = practicing self-compassionate thinking to take the place of our inner critic.
- In our behaviors, self-care = prioritizing time and energy for healthy activities we find enjoyable or relaxing, and setting emotional and interpersonal boundaries to protect our well-being.

Self-care is something that women often put lowest on our list of priorities.

- We stay busy taking care of the needs of our loved ones—our kids, partners, parents—our home, the finances, the cooking, the shopping, work, school . . .
- We tell ourselves, "I am being a good mother/wife/partner/daughter/employee, and I can handle it all."
- There is often little time or energy left to "indulge" in self-care.

But is it indulgence—or is it a necessity? If we spend most of our time taking care of others' needs and the things we "should" do and little to no time taking care of our own needs, we might burn out—get exhausted, depressed, unhealthy, demoralized—and life loses joy.

Self-care starts with an attitude:

- Talking to yourself with self-compassion and not criticism or shaming
- Owning your right to take time for yourself
- Spending time with people who value you and are kind and supportive of you.

Self-care is also about finding a balance in your life, developing a pleasing and optimistic vision of how you would like your life to look, and creating a feasible game plan for how to support those goals:

- It's about taking back control over your life and feeling some freedom about the choices you want to make.
- It means setting aside time to spend on yourself in a wide range of activities that you enjoy and that are emotionally and physically healthy. There are many wellness behaviors, such as exercising; eating healthy foods; not smoking; drinking healthy non-alcoholic beverages; not using illicit drugs; being in nature; enjoying vistas; spending time with people you love and who support you; avoiding toxic people in your life; freeing up time to pursue hobbies, sports, or whatever is relaxing; and carving out time to treat yourself to something nice.
- It involves setting boundaries with people who may otherwise take advantage of you or treat you badly, setting boundaries around taking care of others at your expense, and saying "no" to people or activities you know are not healthy or positive.

Self-Care: Psychological: Self-Care in Our Thoughts (30 minutes)

Have the group follow along with Handout 5.2: Self-Compassion Versus Shame while you review the material and stop occasionally to elicit discussion among the group members (*Does this ring a bell with anyone? Does anyone resonate to the feeling of shame? If so, what do you think your sources of shame might be?*). If possible, link to material you know about particular clients or group themes from prior sessions, and keep an eye out for opportunities to link to alcohol or drug triggers for specific clients in the group.

Next, review Handout 5.3: Self-Care in My Thoughts: Self-Compassion Versus Shame Automatic Thoughts—Sample with the group to teach them what thoughts of self-compassion could be in response to situations that have elicited shame thoughts. Explain the idea of the "self-compassion versus shame" balance in automatic thoughts, and elicit discussion again.

Then, do Exercise 5.1 with a volunteer group member, to model working through Worksheet 5.1: Self-Care in My Thoughts: Self-Compassion Versus Shame Thoughts.

Self-Compassion Versus Shame

What is self-compassion? It means talking to yourself without harsh judgment and criticism, and it leads to more well-being, higher self-esteem, more self-confidence, less anger, and less shame. Practicing self-compassion allows you to feel safe being vulnerable (putting yourself "out there" in relationships and in life, speaking up to say what you want). Self-compassion is an antidote to shame.

Self-compassionate thoughts are very important.

- It matters what you tell yourself. When we fall short or make a mistake, we can talk to ourselves with kindness in the same supportive way we might speak to a friend we care about, rather than berating ourselves in a harsh, critical, judgmental way.
- It is important that you not believe every negative thought about yourself that runs through your head. Don't buy into negative or critical thoughts about yourself. A helpful mindfulness phrase to tell yourself is "Thoughts are not facts." Keep an eye out for negative thoughts. Try to deliberately tell yourself compassionate things and things for which you are grateful.

What is shame? Shame is the experience of feeling flooded with intense painful feelings, such as humiliation and self-loathing, along with beliefs and thoughts that we are damaged and not worthy of being loved, respected, or valued. Red flags of shame are harshly judgmental, self-critical thoughts ("negative self-talk").

What is the difference between shame and guilt? Shame is a global negative reaction *about ourselves* that leaves us with intense feelings of self-loathing. Shame is rarely a useful emotion; it often leads to self-destructive behavior and depression, *not* to positive behavior change. Guilt is a negative reaction about our specific behavior in a certain situation. Guilt is associated with thoughts like, "I did something terrible." Shame is associated with thoughts like, "I am a terrible person. I am a loser. I am disgusting."

Signs of shame can include:

- Flooding of negative emotions (e.g., humiliation, self-loathing)
- Self-destructive behavior (alcohol or drug abuse, cutting)
- Having "no voice"—allowing others to treat us with disrespect, not putting interpersonal boundaries in place to protect our interests, and feeling inadequate to speak up for ourselves

- Low self-esteem
- Judgmental and harshly critical thoughts about ourselves and about others ("I am a failure." "My body is ugly." "No one good will want me." "I have done nothing of importance in my life.")
- Social anxiety and negative social comparison ("I have nothing of value to say here." "These people are better-looking/more accomplished than me.")
- Fear of vulnerability ("If he really knew me, he wouldn't want me. I'd better watch what I say and how I act." "If I speak up, they will know how stupid and incompetent I am.")

Recognize when you are thinking shame thoughts, and learn to treat yourself with self-compassion.

- Notice and track your self-compassion and shame thoughts on the back of your daily monitoring cards each day. Notice which number is higher on a typical day.
- Be on the look-out for "go-to" shame thoughts and try come up with a self-compassion thought when you recognize a shame thought. Practice developing a new "go-to" of self-compassion thoughts in real time. Self-loathing/shame is rarely a useful emotion, and you can work toward freeing yourself from it by focusing on self-compassion thoughts.
- Track trends over time. Are self-compassion thoughts becoming more plentiful? Are shame thoughts less prevalent?

You may have to deliberately remember to ask yourself: What would a self-compassionate thought look like right now? Tell yourself: That's a shame thought—it may feel true, it's what I've been telling myself for years. But is it helpful? Would others think it's true? Can I let it go?

Adapted from Neff & Germer (2018); Brown (2007); Kämmerer (2019)

HANDOUT 5.3
Self-Care in My Thoughts: Self-Compassion Versus Shame
Automatic Thoughts—Sample

Situation	Shame Thought	Self-Compassion Thought
Home alone. I said "no" to going out for dinner with friends in my efforts to avoid alcohol triggers.	I am such a loser, can't even go out with my friends.	I'm doing the more difficult, but right thing; this is the less risky path. I'll make myself a cranberry ice and watch a movie. The cravings will go away if I don't drink. I'm on the right track.
I bought a bottle of wine and drank alone at home.	I am a failure. I will never get better. If I vanished, the world would be a better place.	I can do this. Throw out the rest of the bottle and go to sleep. I'm making progress and this is really hard. Tomorrow morning I'll feel better than I do now.
Waking up early, can't fall back to sleep, feeling depressed	I'm an idiot. I just let my life go by and put up with way too much. I've wasted 20 years.	I've made mistakes in my life like everyone, but I am a loving person and I have helped many people. My family is lucky to have me.
After a date that didn't go well	I am broken inside. He must have been smart enough to see that.	Not every date goes well. It just wasn't a good match. When I find the right person, I'll know it.
At a work meeting	They seem to value me here. They don't know what a mess I am or they wouldn't have hired me.	Oh, this must be that "imposter syndrome"—feeling as though I'm not as competent as I actually am. I'm not going to fall for it. I have a solid education and years of experience, and I'm going to embrace this positive feedback.

EXERCISE 5.1
Self-Care: Self-Compassion in Thoughts

In this exercise, clients will practice labeling automatic thoughts as either shame-based or self-compassionate, to learn to identify and replace shame thoughts with self-compassion self-talk. Using the flipchart/whiteboard, work with a volunteer to think of and write down situations that elicit shame thoughts in response. Then help the volunteer replace shame thoughts with self-compassion thoughts for each situation, while the rest of group watches, provides input/ideas, and writes their own thoughts down on their worksheets. After that, open up the session for group-wide discussion (*What did others write down for your automatic self-compassion or shame thoughts? How did it feel to do this exercise? Can anyone share one thing you learned about yourself from this exercise?*).

WORKSHEET 5.1

Self-Care in My Thoughts: Self-Compassion Versus Shame Automatic Thoughts

Situation	Shame Thought	Self-Compassion Thought

EXERCISE 5.2
Self-Care: Behavioral—Habits for Well-Being Brainstorm and Schedule Self-Care Activities to Create Habits for Well-Being (15 minutes)

Discuss the importance of deliberately planning and scheduling self-care behaviors on a regular basis, using Handout 5.4: Self-Care in My Habits for Well-Being: Behaviors— Sample to provide examples of self-care, and then enlist a volunteer group member to work through Worksheet 5.2: Self-Care in My Habits for Well-Being: Behaviors with you, using the flipchart and having the other group members follow along and contribute ideas and reactions while also starting to fill out their own Worksheet 5.2. Then, open for discussion, asking other group members to share what habits for well-being they came up with.

Also note that self-care is *not* the same as being selfish. Self-care typically refers to tending to the well-being and happiness of oneself *and* often to one's family as well; taking care of others can often be a healthy and desirable activity.

Brainstorm and Schedule Self-Care Activities to Create Habits for Well-Being

Using Worksheet 5.2: Self-Care in My Habits for Well-Being: Behaviors, ask for a volunteer to work with you (use the flipchart) to think of and write down self-care activities the volunteer can do this week and/ or this month. Have other group members follow along to complete their own Worksheet 5.2, while also contributing to discussion around the volunteer's list.

HANDOUT 5.4
Self-Care in My Habits for Well-Being: Behaviors—Sample

What I Do Now	What I Want to Do Going Forward	Scheduled?
Try to avoid sugar	Continue avoiding sugar but add more green vegetables and fiber to diet. Also eat fish twice a week	
Eat ice cream twice a week	Eat ice cream once every 2 weeks	
Don't enjoy the kids much	Spend more pleasant time with the kids, go to park, watch them laugh	Yes, movie time and park this week
Skip church	Go to church each week—it makes me feel connected and good	Yes
Skip annual physical	See primary care doctor for annual exam	Yes
Do yoga class once a week	Continue	Yes
Walk maybe once a week	Brisk walk every other day, half a mile, with the kids and/or Jim sometimes	Yes, when wake up
Like to swim but don't make the time	Swim once a week	Saturday morning
Mani/pedi once a month	Continue, ask Sasha if she wants to come with	Yes
Hard time saying "no"	Say "no" at least 2 times/month to my sister who asks me to babysit my niece every week	
Hard time speaking up about Jim's family visits	Tell Jim he needs to consult with me before inviting his family over	
No daily "down time"	Leave time before bed each night to relax and read or watch TV, and/or relax with Jim and the kids	Yes
Not much social support	Go to meetings at least twice a week (schedule with Jim; get babysitter if need to)	Yes, 2x/week
See therapist once a week	Continue	Yes
See psychiatrist once a month	Continue	Yes

WORKSHEET 5.2

Self-Care in My Habits for Well-Being: Behaviors

What I Do Now	What I Want to Do Going Forward	Scheduled?

EXERCISE 5.3
Self-Care: Behavioral Want/Should Balance in My Lifestyle (15 minutes)

Begin this next section as follows:

Lifestyle balance is about being healthy and content—having the right balance of time spent doing responsibilities/work activities, leisure activities, and self-care activities, as well as spending time with people who are healthy, supportive, kind, and important to you. Giving up alcohol and drugs (which take time, energy, attention, and money) frees you up to use newfound time to things you should do and things you want to do.

In this exercise, clients will look at how well they are balancing their "shoulds" with their "wants" and then think about how they might rebalance those "shoulds" and "wants" to promote well-being. They will be using Handout 5.5: Lifestyle Want/Should Balance Worksheet—Sample and Worksheet 5.3: Lifestyle Want/Should Balance Worksheet.

After reviewing Handout 5.5 with them, ask for a volunteer to work with you (using the flipchart) to fill in the left column of Worksheet 5.3 (i.e., activities she does in a typical week that are her "shoulds"). Then, have her complete the middle column on the worksheet, what she might "want" to do during her week. You may have to discuss/ brainstorm how to reduce some time the volunteer spends doing her "shoulds" or other activities (some unwanted, such as drinking/using drugs/passed out/intoxicated) in order to make time to do some of her "wants." Be realistic: There are only so many hours in the week. Help her consider delegating some of her "shoulds" to others, and/or eliminating or minimizing some of her "shoulds" that, upon reconsideration, may feel less important to her—for instance, not preparing a different specific food for each family member every night, or not vacuuming the house daily. Help challenge some perfection beliefs that many women have ("I need to be the perfect mother/wife, etc."). You may have to discuss saying "no" to spending some time helping a family member or friend in order to redirect that time to spend on herself.

Have other group members follow along to complete their own Worksheet 5.3, while contributing to the discussion around the volunteer's work on the want/should balance. Expect some resistance to reducing the time or number of "should" activities; use a non-confrontational, motivational interviewing approach to help the women understand that their own self-care is very important and worth prioritizing. Also, point out that the time previously spent drinking or using drugs is now free to fill with a healthy balance of "want" and "should" activities.

Lifestyle Want/Should Balance Worksheet—Sample

- We all do a lot of different things each week. Some of us spend almost all of our time doing what we "should" do and not enough of what we "want" to do—we don't have enough self-care activities.
- Alcohol and drug use take time away from both shoulds and wants. Count the number of hours you spent in a typical week drinking/using drugs, being intoxicated/high, or being passed out. If you no longer do these things, the hours are "found time" to replace with both shoulds and wants in your schedule.
- The table below shows a list of the things a person might do in a typical week, along with the percent of time doing them. Each activity is listed in either the "should" list or the "want" list. Not all "shoulds" are unwanted—you may enjoy and value them. Some shoulds are also wants (note those in your table).
- Then, figure out how to rearrange your weekly schedule to add in more "want" activities—use the blank want/should balance worksheet page.

"Should"		"Want"	
Activity	**Current/ Adjusted Hours in Week**	**Activity**	**Current/ Adjusted Hours in Week**
Work (also a want)	25	Hanging out with partner	2/6
Commute	8	Hanging out with kids/family	4/6
Housework	6/4	Riding bike	0/1
Garden work (also a want)	2-5	Gym, swim	0/3
Errands	3	Go out to the movies	1x/month
Driving kids around	10/6	Go out to eat	1x/week
Food shopping/cooking (like to cook)	10/8	Vacations	2x/year
Paying bills	2	Be outside with dog, walk	2-3
		See my friends	0x/1x week
		Relax and read a novel/watch TV	4/6

WORKSHEET 5.3
Lifestyle Want/Should Balance Worksheet

"Should"		"Want"	
Activity	Current/Adjusted Hours in Week	Activity	Current/Adjusted Hours in Week

Farewell to Members Leaving the Group (10 minutes)

Have members who are leaving identify the skills they think have been most important to the changes that they have made during therapy—that is, those skills they will continue to try to implement in order to maintain their progress. Remind group members that relapses most often occur in the types of situations they are now prepared to handle.

For women finishing the group, ask them how they feel about finishing the treatment program. Explore termination issues—fear, relief, loss. Discuss referrals for additional treatment if necessary. Discuss the possibility that group members may wish to stay in contact and provide support to one another.

Each group member who is finishing treatment should also be asked to go around the room and say something positive or constructive to each of her fellow group members. These statements could focus on positive changes or steps the leaving group member has seen each of the other women make during treatment, or ways in which the leaving group member feels she herself has learned or benefited from other women in the group. Other group members also should be encouraged to give some positive feedback to the woman who is finishing treatment. Women who are finishing treatment and the therapist may also want to say something to one another.

Anticipating High-Risk Situations This Week (5 minutes)

Rationale:

At the end of each session, we will spend a bit of time discussing any problem situations that each member thinks might come up around drinking or drug use this week. As you each progress through therapy, you will get better and better at anticipating and handling these. A "high-risk situation" is a situation in which you would find it very difficult not to drink. Today, I'd like us each to spend a few minutes together thinking about the upcoming week. [For each group member:] Are there any situations that you might encounter this week that would tempt you to drink or use drugs

EXERCISE 5.4
High-Risk Situations and Executing High-Risk Situation Plans

Use Worksheet 5.4: High-Risk Situations, located in the Client Workbook:

Now let's each use Worksheet 5.4: High-Risk Situations to write in a high-risk situation for this upcoming week and brainstorm together about strategies/solutions you can use to cope with that high-risk situation in order to avoid drinking or using drugs in response to it. Are there any situations that you might encounter this week that would tempt you to drink or use drugs?

Elicit examples of upcoming high-risk situations from members and brainstorm together to generate plans for how to handle the situation for two or three group members. Write ideas about how to handle this situation on the High-Risk Situations worksheet. Refer to Session 1 in this guide for a copy of the worksheet or to the Client Workbook.

Assign Homework (5 minutes)

Here is a list of homework assignments for each group member to complete between today's session and the next. Remind the women how important it is to complete the homework.

1. Complete one self-monitoring card each day.
2. On the back of your self-monitoring cards, write down high-risk situations you encountered and how you handled those.
3. Continue daily review of the 3×5 card from the decisional matrix (Worksheet 4.2: My Positive and Negative Consequences Reminder Card).
4. Read all the Session 5 material in your workbook and complete worksheets you didn't finish during the session.
5. Complete Worksheet 5.4: High-Risk Situations, located in the Client Workbook, and execute high-risk situation plans.

CHAPTER 11

Session 6: Identifying Anxiety, Depression, Trauma; Coping with Cravings

(Corresponds to Chapter 6 in the Client Workbook)

(1.5 hours)

Notes to the Therapist Before the Session

1. For rolling-admission groups (see Chapter 3), each new member should have an individual assessment (see Chapter 5) with the group facilitator prior to joining the group. At the end of the assessment session, for women joining the group at any session (i.e., Session 2–12) after Session 1, the therapist should spend an additional 30 minutes with each new group member to provide the Client Workbook and to review basic information covered in Session 1 that the client will need to know to proceed with all subsequent sessions. This includes coverage of use of the Client Workbook and group rules, as well as a brief review of core treatment elements, including self-monitoring, psychoeducation, high-risk situations, triggers, and behavior chains (see Session 2). That way, no matter what session the new member is entering, she will be able to do daily self-monitoring and understand the basics of high-risk situations, triggers, and behavior chains.

2. Each rolling-admission group session with a new member starts with a 5-minute round robin introduction of each group member, and 10 minutes of assessment feedback to the new member(s) (see Session 1 for detailed instructions and feedback sheets). Members in the group at different stages of recovery can provide support to the new client and share their own feedback from their first session. If a new member is lacking relevant information from previous sessions, she can review sessions in the Client Workbook or you can briefly describe the

section, and/or abstinent members can be encouraged to spend time with the new member after session to explain relevant prior material.

3. For each new member entering the group in Sessions 2 to 12, follow instructions at the beginning of each session regarding Introductions and Providing Assessment Feedback in Client's First Session.

4. If this is a client's first session, you must summarize data from the pretreatment assessment to fill in a Feedback Sheet (see Handout 1.10 in Client Workbook) for each client in the group in preparation for her first session.

5. Before the session begins, write the session agenda on a flipchart, whiteboard, or blackboard.

6. If you are doing the Optional Graphing Intervention, see instructions in Chapter 3 of this Therapist Guide.

7. All worksheets and handouts used in this treatment program appear in this Therapist Guide and in the corresponding Client Workbook; worksheets (and selected handouts) can also be accessed by searching for this book's title on the Oxford Academic platform, at academic. oup.com.

Session 6 Outline

All times are approximate and should be adjusted based on clinical need and whether group time needs to be devoted to new or departing members.

1. Pre-session sign-in and substance use check (15 minutes before session begins)
2. Introductions and agenda setting (5 minutes)
3. Check-in, review of self-monitoring and homework (10 minutes)
4. What is anxiety? (15 minutes)
5. What is depression? (15 minutes)
6. What is trauma? (15 minutes)
7. Coping with cravings to drink or use Drugs (20 minutes)
8. Farewell to members leaving the group (10 minutes)
9. Anticipating high-risk situations this week (5 minutes)
10. Assign homework (5 minutes)

1. Flipchart, whiteboard, or blackboard, felt-tip markers or chalk, eraser
2. Breathalyzer and tubes or saliva strips (optional)
3. Saliva drug tests for each group member (optional)
4. Seven self-monitoring cards for each group member (Note to therapist: Keep a stack of these to give group members at each session.)
5. OPTIONAL: Individualized graph for each woman
6. Handouts
    6.1: The Relationship Between Anxiety, Depression, and Alcohol/Drugs: Get Off the Roller Coaster!
    6.2: What Is a Craving to Use Drugs or Alcohol?
    6.3: Tips to Cope with Cravings for Alcohol/Drugs
    6.4: Coping with Cravings: Sample Worksheet
7. Worksheets
    6.1: Taking Stock of Your Anxiety
    6.2: What Do You Get Anxious About?
    6.3: What Do You Get Depressed About?
    6.4: Figuring Out Your Trauma Symptoms
    6.5: How Trauma Symptoms and Drinking/Drugs Interact
    6.6: Coping with Cravings
    6.7: High-Risk Situations [See Client Workbook Worksheet 6.7]

Pre-Session Sign-In and Substance Use Check (15 minutes pre-session)

If any member of the group appears to be high or intoxicated, you may want to assess her blood alcohol level (BAL) with a breathalyzer or saliva strip or use a saliva drug screen. Regardless of formal testing, though, if a group member is visibly high or intoxicated, review the treatment agreement with her and let her know that she will not be allowed to attend this session. Clients who miss a session will not receive a make-up session, but encourage them to read the handouts they missed for that session and complete the homework for the following week. You should assist the client in arranging alternate transportation home, review her abstinence plan, and remind her of her abstinence goal.

Introductions and Agenda Setting (5 minutes)

You will introduce new members joining the group this session, and provide an overview (i.e., set agenda) of what will be covered in the session. The purpose of Session 6 is (1) to discuss the prevalence of anxiety, depression, and trauma as common mental health issues among women with substance use disorder and (2) to identify symptoms and experiences of anxiety, depression, and trauma. Clients will learn more about cravings to drink/use drugs and strategies to handle cravings. Ask the group if there is anything pressing they would like to discuss today. Explain the absence of missing members without revealing protected health information.

Check-In, Review of Self-Monitoring and Homework (10 minutes)

Check-in follows a "round robin" format, in which drinking status and homework are emphasized. To introduce the round robin check-in:

We're going to go around the room using what we call a "round robin check-in" to get a brief version of how your week has been, focusing on your alcohol use, drug use, cravings, and triggers; how you coped with triggers and cravings; in hindsight what you might have done differently (with therapist and group input/ideas as well); homework you completed and what was helpful about it. We also will answer or clarify any questions or concerns about the homework material. Each group member will have a few minutes [depending on how many women there are in the group] *to discuss with the group how your coping with alcohol/drug use triggers has been this week.*

> **Therapist Note**
> *Try to pay particular attention to women's specific themes (e.g., right to self-care, empowerment) to link experiences to the specific theme: "One theme I've heard that's common among several of you is . . ."*

Go around the room and ask each group member how her week was (focusing on alcohol and/or drug use); listen while looking over her self-monitoring cards; and link what she is saying to her daily cards for alcohol/drug cravings, triggers, and use. Use information from this for specific topics in the rest of the session. Check in with each group member and discuss the progress of her abstinence plan. Update the plan if necessary. Also remember to ask each client at the end of her round robin time about what homework she was able to complete.

You should reinforce self-recording behavior, check for questions or problems, and help group members develop solutions for difficulties related to self-recording procedures. Ask members if they have any questions. Possible questions to anticipate include:

- **Question:** I thought about drinking the whole morning. Is that one urge or more than one?

THERAPIST: *You had the urge continually?*
CLIENT: Not every minute.
THERAPIST: *Well, each time you have a thought or an image about having a specific type of drink or a drink in a particular situation, that counts as a separate urge. Can you share some specific situations you thought about?*

- **Question:** Why are my urges so much higher than everyone else's? Why am I the only one still drinking?

THERAPIST: *It's natural that you would want to compare your drinking/ drug use and urges to those of the other group members. Although this can be an important motivator, it also is important to remember that everyone has her own unique path to abstinence. You're working on it, so be patient with yourself, and think of the changes you've already made! What does the group think about what _____ said?*

Therapist Note
After reviewing the daily monitoring cards, for outpatient settings you may wish to include the optional Graphing Intervention here.

Optional Graphing Intervention for Outpatient Treatment Settings

See the detailed instructions in Chapter 3 of this guide for how to use the graphs located in Session 2 of the Therapist Guide and in the Client Workbook (Handout 2.1. Graph: Alcohol/Drug Use and Urges

Sample. Graph: Alcohol/Drug Use and Urges). This intervention will allow each woman to track her progress by entering weekly data summarized from her daily monitoring cards: 1. Number of drinks; 2. Number of drugs used; 3. Number of urges/cravings; and 4. Average strength of urges/cravings.

Other Homework Review

Review all other homework clients did during the prior week. Reinforce clients for completing homework and discuss barriers experienced in completing the homework. Ask questions such as, *"What did you learn from the homework?"* or *"How can you use the homework to help you in the future?"*

Remember that as part of homework review, each week you need to review group members' recording of high-risk situations and how these were handled: *"Who wants to share how you handled one of your high-risk situations this week without drinking/using drugs?"* Elicit high-risk examples from two or three group members and get feedback from other members. Remember to have group members direct their comments to the other group members, and not just to you. Point out common types of high-risk situations among the group members and encourage women facing similar situations to share how they coped or ideas for coping. Selectively model and repeat empowering and motivational positive affirmations that group members give to one another: for example, *"We know this is hard, you're doing great." "Next time you'll be able to use a different strategy, hang in there."*

Also, ask about progress with doctor's appointments and blood tests. Due to time constraints, group members should discuss any concerns about their blood test or feedback with you after the group. Ask each client to bring in a copy of her lab results and give it to you. You can give feedback to the client during review of homework either that week or the week after.

Share the following with the group:

The time in the treatment group is only part of the process. The real change occurs when you practice changing your lives in the real world. The group will help you get ideas, stay motivated, keep you on track, and develop an understanding of the problem. But actually changing behavior takes place in your everyday life—at home, at work, with family, friends, and so on.

Group members who are having substantial difficulty with their abstinence plan or who appear to be at risk for an emergency should be asked discreetly to remain after group for an individual check-in with you.

What Is Anxiety? (15 minutes)

As you review the rationale for Exercise 6.1: What Is Anxiety? refer group members to Handout 6.1: The Relationship Between Anxiety, Depression, and Alcohol/Drugs: Get Off the Roller Coaster! and Worksheets 6.1: Taking Stock of Your Anxiety, and 6.2: What Do You Get Anxious About?

Overall Rationale for Anxiety, Depression, and Trauma:

Women, especially problem drinkers and drug users, tend to struggle with anxiety and sadness in their lives, and many also have experienced lasting effects of traumatic events in their lives. Today we will discuss and determine if and how anxiety, depression, and/or trauma affect you, and how they might relate to your alcohol/drug use. These negative emotional states tend to be common triggers for women to drink/use drugs—alcohol/drugs may be used as a coping strategy to reduce or avoid strong negative emotions. Drinking or using drugs may work in the very short term, but almost inevitably makes things worse overall. Next week, we'll follow up with some new sober strategies to help you to handle strong negative emotions and to calm yourself. You can use these new coping skills in the face of strong negative emotions that might in the past have been a trigger to drink or use drugs.

Let's talk about anxiety first.

Most people experience some level of anxiety at some points in their lives. It's a normal human emotion that is "hard-wired" in all animals, designed to warn us of danger. In some situations, low levels of anxiety can actually improve your performance. For instance, when taking a test in school, a bit of anxiety can help you to concentrate on the test. High levels of anxiety, however, are usually counterproductive, making it harder to focus on the task at hand. Anxiety has cognitive (thoughts) components and also has physiological components such as elevated heart rate and release of stress hormones and stimulating chemicals to activate our bodies and prepare us for a "fight, flight, or freeze" response to perceived danger. Many types of anxiety experienced by humans these days are mostly "false alarms"—that is, our brains and bodies are activated to protect us against a perceived threat or danger that is actually just triggered from prior experiences or beliefs; we are usually not actually in danger. High levels of anxiety are extremely uncomfortable and can be disabling.

If you suspect you suffer from anxiety more than the average person, we should discuss it to determine if additional treatment might be helpful. If you feel that anxiety is not a big problem for you, I think you will still benefit from learning how to manage everyday feelings of anxiety.

EXERCISE 6.1
What Is Anxiety?

Generate discussion using Worksheets 6.1: Taking Stock of Your Anxiety and 6.2: What Do You Get Anxious About? as guides. Discuss group members' experiences of anxiety and the types of situations that generate anxiety for them. During this discussion, ask group members to begin filling out Worksheet 6.2 in their workbooks, which they should complete for homework.

WORKSHEET 6.1
Taking Stock of Your Anxiety

These are some common anxiety symptoms. Put a ✓ next to ones you have experienced.

▪ **Breathing/Chest Symptoms**
Shortness of breath
Rapid or shallow breathing
Pressure on chest
Lump in throat
Choking sensations

▪ **Skin-Related Symptoms**
Sweating
Hot and cold spells
Itching

▪ **Heart/Blood Pressure Symptoms**
Heart racing
Palpitations
Faintness
Increased/decreased blood pressure

▪ **Behavioral Symptoms**
Avoidance
Irritability
Compulsive, repetitive acts

▪ **Intestinal Symptoms**
Loss of appetite
Nausea or vomiting
Stomach discomfort

▪ **Muscular Symptoms**
Shaking, tremors
Eyelid twitching
Upper back and/or neck tension
Startle reactions
Pacing

▪ **Cognitive/Emotional Symptoms**
Intrusive thoughts
Nightmares
Depersonalization (feeling outside of yourself)
Brief hallucinations
Paranoia and fear
Obsessing with no relief
Worry about everyday events
Insomnia

Which ones have you experienced, and when?

_____

_____

What have you done to try to get relief?

_____

_____

_____

Adapted in part from *How to Control Your Anxiety Before It Controls You* (Ellis, 1995).

WORKSHEET 6.2
What Do You Get Anxious About?

These are some common types of anxiety. Put a ✓ next to ones you have experienced.

■ **Social Anxiety**
Socializing
Public speaking
Job-related activities
Being the center of attention

■ **Specific Phobias**
Open places/closed places
Flying
Heights
Trains, bridges, tunnels
Animals, insects

■ **Generalized Anxiety: Thoughts About . . .**
Things that could go wrong
Not being able to pay the bills
People I love getting hurt

■ **Obsessions/Compulsions**
Intrusive thoughts; Feeling very detached
Fear of germs; Fear of hurting others
Fear of being bad; Checking for safety

■ **Panic Attacks**
Being nervous about having another panic attack

■ **Post-Traumatic Stress**
Exposure to something that reminds me of the trauma (alone at night, etc.)
Flashbacks and memories of traumatic experiences, nightmares
Feeling vulnerable, unsafe
Feeling numb, unloving
Feeling irritable

What do you get anxious about?

_____

_____

How do you feel when you're anxious?

_____

_____

What works to make you feel less anxious?

_____

_____

What Is Depression? (15 minutes)

Distribute Worksheet 6.3: What Do You Get Depressed About? to group members while reading the rationale for Exercise 6.2: What Is Depression?

Rationale:

Another common problem among female problem drinkers is depression and sadness. We all feel sad from time to time. Passing feelings of sadness or depression are normal and common. Like anxiety and trauma, feelings of sadness and depression can be triggers to drink or use drugs excessively, and, like anxiety, depression is usually made worse in the long run by excessive drinking or drug use. So, it's important for women who drink or use drugs to be aware of their moods, and to be able to change their moods through methods that do not involve alcohol or drugs.

EXERCISE 6.2
What Is Depression?

In this exercise, you will help clients to look at common symptoms of depression and identify which and how specific symptoms affect each client. Use Handout 6.1: The Relationship Between Anxiety, Depression, and Alcohol/Drugs: Get Off the Roller Coaster! and Worksheet 6.3: What Do You Get Depressed About?

> *Let's look at whether sadness and depression have been problematic in your lives, and then we'll follow up next week with some tips on how to manage negative moods.*
>
> *While we talk about whether you have struggled with sadness or depression, let's use Worksheet: 6.3: What Do You Get Depressed About? to identify symptoms of depression you may have been experiencing recently. Then, we'll talk about what types of situations have made you feel depressed in the past so that we can figure out how you can cope with these situations without drinking or using drugs. Remember, drinking or drug use may be a short-term solution to escape feelings of sadness and depression, but in the long run, it makes the depression worse and also creates a new set of problems that themselves can cause you to get depressed. Let's find a way out of the vicious cycle. You can finish filling in the worksheet for homework this week.*

Generate discussion using Worksheet 6.3 as a guide. Discuss group members' experiences of depression and what types of situations generate depression for them. Highlight shared experiences and link to women's issues around alcohol and depression.

At the end of this discussion, you should reiterate to the group the connection between depression/anxiety and drinking/drug use, using Handout 6.1. Also provide psychoeducation that benzodiazepines (e.g., Valium, Xanax, Ativan, Klonopin) are likely to have the same "vicious cycle" relationship with anxiety and depression that alcohol does. You can also point out that the hallmark symptom of cocaine withdrawal is a steep crash into deep depression, which also sets up people to seek temporary relief by using cocaine again. And with marijuana, the vicious cycle is more about irritability, depression, and restlessness after marijuana leaves the system.

WORKSHEET 6.3
What Do You Get Depressed About?

These are some common symptoms of depression:

- Depressed mood
- Sadness
- Apathy
- Being tearful
- Feeling empty
- Thoughts of death, thoughts of suicide
- Decreased interest in things you used to enjoy
- Sleeping more than usual or unable to sleep
- Feeling worthless, low self-esteem
- Fatigue or loss of energy
- Feelings of hopelessness
- Waking up at 4 or 5 am ruminating on hopeless, self-loathing thoughts
- Difficulty concentrating (hard to read newspaper, book)
- Change in appetite
- Moving slowly, as if under water

What situations tend to make you feel depressed?

_____

_____

What thoughts tend to make you feel depressed?

_____

_____

How do you feel when you are depressed?

_____

_____

What works to make you feel less depressed?

_____

_____

The Relationship Between Anxiety, Depression, and Alcohol/Drugs: Get Off the Roller Coaster!

Alcohol, anxiety, and depression:

- Alcohol depresses (slows down) your central nervous system, but it tricks you first!
- *In the short run,* alcohol makes you feel euphoric, happy, and relaxed.
- However, when the alcohol increases in your system to a certain point, it can make you feel depressed, irritable, and/or angry.
- When the alcohol leaves your system, *the withdrawal effects are opposite those of the initial effects.* That is, you feel a "rebound effect" of anxiety—you're even more anxious! You also may feel depressed, irritable, and restless.
- In other words, the use of alcohol *temporarily* (and artificially) erases the negative feelings (anxiety, depression) that made you want to drink in the first place, but then it actually *magnifies* (increases) the very same anxiety and depressive symptoms that made you want to drink or use. Now you feel even more anxious and depressed—which makes you feel like you need to drink again to get rid of those feelings again.
- *It's a vicious cycle.* When experiencing the increased anxiety/depression withdrawal symptoms after alcohol use, it's common for people to think, "Wow, I must be really anxious (depressed)—even more than I thought. If I don't have alcohol in my system, I feel REALLY anxious. I'd better have a drink to calm my nerves again and get rid of this awful anxiety (prevent another panic attack, stop these obsessive thoughts)."
- Many people don't realize that it's actually the *alcohol* that is causing an increase in the anxiety or depression!
- The only way to stop this vicious cycle is to *get off the roller coaster*—stop drinking and learn to cope with the anxiety and depression that led you to drink in the first place. Longer-term solutions take time to learn and practice. *You have to tolerate a certain amount of discomfort while you are learning to control your anxiety and depression without alcohol or drugs.*
- There are non-addictive antidepressant and anti-anxiety medications available to help as well.

Other drugs, anxiety, and depression:

- Ask your therapist about the similar "vicious cycle" or "roller coaster" relationships among other substances (e.g., benzodiazepines, marijuana, cocaine, stimulants), withdrawal symptoms, and relapse.
- Benzodiazepines (Valium, Xanax, Ativan, and so on) operate in the same way, but even more intensely and more destructively than alcohol.
- Marijuana withdrawal causes irritability, depression, and restlessness, which set up cravings to use it again for temporary relief.
- Cocaine withdrawal is associated with sudden and severe depression.
- Stimulant withdrawal is associated with depression, irritability, and fatigue.

It is important to know that heavy drinking or drug use interferes with the effectiveness of most antidepressants that your doctor prescribes, so you need to stop drinking or using other drugs to let your depression or anxiety medication take effect.

What Is Trauma? (15 minutes)

You may introduce this material as follows:

Trauma symptoms or a full-blown post-traumatic stress disorder (PTSD) can develop after experiencing or witnessing first-hand a traumatic, often life-threatening event, such as an assault or rape, an accident, combat, or a natural disaster. Trauma symptoms often result in avoidance of things that remind you of the trauma, and they can interfere with your interpersonal relationships and enjoyment of life.

You may feel like you are on edge, as if you are living in constant danger. Or common things, such as when someone is yelling or is angry, may trigger trauma reactions linked to a history of assault that happened even 20 years ago, or longer. Alcohol and drug use problems are common in PTSD, because people sometimes use these substances to help avoid or escape unpleasant memories, to relax, or to sleep without nightmares.

There is also "betrayal trauma" in which someone, who you may have counted on to protect, you actually put you in danger or did not protect you from danger or abuse.

If relevant to group members, you should review with the group Worksheet 6.4: Figuring Out Your Trauma Symptoms, and Worksheet 6.5: How Trauma Symptoms and Drinking/Drugs Interact, and elicit discussion—*What rings a bell here for anyone?* Look for and highlight shared experiences and themes, and reiterate the importance of self-care and self-compassion. Note that some cognitive behavioral therapy techniques will be presented in Session 7 to help regulate strong negative emotions.

EXERCISE 6.3
What Is Trauma?

Read through Worksheets 6.4: Figuring Out Your Trauma Symptoms and 6.5: How Trauma Symptoms and Drinking/Drugs Interact, while having group members begin filling in their individual worksheets. Do not have a volunteer model this exercise with you; instead, encourage group discussion while you read through the worksheets and stop to have group members complete parts of them in the course of discussion.

While we discuss these worksheets, feel free to fill out yours and share with the group what you are thinking of writing or what you wrote. Give each other support, feedback, and ideas.

WORKSHEET 6.4
Figuring Out Your Trauma Symptoms

Circle each of the post-traumatic stress disorder (PTSD) symptoms you have experienced, and put a star next to any that are troublesome to you.

Intrusive Re-Experiencing of Symptoms

- Painful memories of the traumatic event
- Nightmares related to the traumatic event
- Suddenly acting or feeling as if the traumatic event is happening again
- Feeling as if you are detached from yourself and/or watching yourself from afar
- Feeling intense distress in response to things that remind you of the trauma
- Increased physical arousal (heartbeat, sweating, shaking, on edge) in response to things that remind you of the trauma

Avoidance of Reminders of the Trauma

- Efforts to avoid thoughts, feelings, situations, activities, or emotions that trigger memories of the trauma

Negative Changes in Thoughts and Mood

- Cannot remember aspects of the trauma
- Negative beliefs and expectations about yourself or the world after the trauma (The world is not safe; I am never safe)
- Blame of self or others for causing the traumatic event (If only I had. . . the trauma event would not have happened)
- Frequent negative trauma-related feelings such as horror, shame, fear
- Less interest or engagement in activities that used to feel important
- Feeling detached, numb, not caring about others
- Difficulty feeling positive emotions

Changes in Arousal and Reactivity

- Frequent irritability or anger
- Impulsive risky or self-destructive behavior
- Hypervigilance (always scanning for or on edge for possible danger)
- Startling easily in response to loud or unexpected noises or situations
- Difficulty concentrating
- Difficulty sleeping

Adapted from American Psychiatric Association (2013)

WORKSHEET 6.5
How Trauma Symptoms and Drinking/Drug Use Interact

Trauma, Alcohol, and Drugs

More than half of women seeking alcohol or drug treatment also have post-traumatic stress disorder (PTSD). There are many reasons why the two disorders occur together:

- Women who have experienced traumas may use alcohol or other substances to manage PTSD symptoms such as irritability, feeling "keyed up," and having difficulty sleeping.
- Substance use can lead to risky behaviors and unintended victimization in traumatic situations.
- Alcohol and drug use can make PTSD symptoms worse over time, which may lead the trauma survivor to drink or use drugs even more—it can become a vicious circle.

Why Women with PTSD or Trauma Use Alcohol and Drugs

- Women living with PTSD or trauma symptoms are often living with physical or mental pain, have difficult and/or shameful memories and dreams they wish to avoid, feel cut-off from others, and have nightmares that interrupt sleep. It makes sense that they would want to find some ways to relax and feel better, even if it is only temporary.
- Alcohol and drugs become a way to deal with sleep problems and feeling uncomfortable "in their own skin."
- Women with PTSD or a trauma history often suffer deep shame as a result of trauma such as sexual assault, and drinking can provide them temporary relief.
- Women with sexual assault or medical trauma may drink or use drugs to feel relaxed enough to have sexual relations.

Interplay of PTSD or Trauma and Alcohol/Drug Symptoms

- Sometimes it can be difficult to tell which symptoms are from PTSD and which are from alcohol/drug problems, since experiences such as insomnia, irritability, self-blame or guilt, negative emotions, or feeling alienated from others can be caused by PTSD or substance use.
- Also, trauma symptoms can trigger substance use, and vice versa. Research suggests that PTSD symptoms can actually increase substance cravings.
- Thus, women with trauma who are working to reduce their substance use may need to develop strategies to manage their PTSD symptoms if they are going to be successful in becoming abstinent. For example, for sleep problems from trauma symptoms, using "sleep hygiene" strategies, rather than alcohol, for insomnia may be helpful. Having a plan to cope with PTSD symptoms may help to reduce or eliminate use of alcohol or drugs to self-medicate trauma symptoms.

There are effective treatments for PTSD or trauma symptoms that you may decide to seek out after or concurrent with dealing with your alcohol/drug problem.

In the spaces below, list up to three trauma symptoms that may be impacting your alcohol/drug use, and your initial coping plan for them:

1. Symptom _____

   Coping Plan _____

2. Symptom _____

   Coping Plan _____

3. Symptom _____

   Coping Plan _____

Describe one way you think reducing your alcohol/drug use will help you manage your trauma symptoms:

_____

_____

_____

_____

Adapted with permission from Shirley Glynn, Ph.D. (see Sautter et al. 2011, 2015).

Rationale:

When people have a drinking or drug habit, or when they cut down or stop using drugs/alcohol, it is natural and expected that they will experience cravings (sometimes called urges) to drink/use drugs. This differs for everyone, but it's not unusual for cravings to be quite intense for the first days or weeks, then continue, but gradually become less frequent and weaker over the next few weeks/months. Cravings can resurface even after that—on anniversaries of stressful events, for instance, or anniversaries of stopping use—or in trigger situations or during stressful times.

It is important that you understand what a craving is and what it means (or doesn't mean), so that you can be in a better position to cope with cravings in ways other than drinking or using drugs.

Ask the following questions to help the group members articulate and discuss their own beliefs about urges and counter these beliefs where appropriate:

I'd like to discuss some of your understanding of cravings to drink/use drugs by asking you some questions, and then we'll work on ways to help you cope with urges to drink/use drugs. First: Where do you think that cravings come from? Second: What do you think it means if you are experiencing cravings/urges?

Therapist Note

Here you should try to help group members view urges as signs of the need to cope with a situation differently, not as a signal to use. Also, help the group members to view urges as time-limited.

EXERCISE 6.4
Understand Cravings: How to Recognize Cravings
and What Does a Craving Mean?

We will go over some information on cravings so you can think about them in a helpful way. We will also briefly review some strategies/tips for coping with cravings.

Review Handout 6.2: What Is a Craving to Use Drugs or Alcohol? and then review Handout 6.3: Tips to Cope with Cravings for Alcohol/Drugs. Elicit a bit of discussion with the group after each handout: *Any thoughts? What might you utilize going forward from this information we just heard?*

Workon and discuss Handout 6.4: Coping with Cravings: Sample Worksheet, with the group via group discussion, while each woman completes her own Worksheet 6.6: Coping with Cravings. Have the women share ideas with the group, brainstorm together, suggest tweaks to their strategies, etc. Lead the discussion with specific suggestions/questions.

HANDOUT 6.2
What Is a Craving to Use Drugs or Alcohol?

Cravings to drink/use drugs are *thoughts* (e.g., "A glass of wine would taste great right now"; "I really need to get high") or *physical feelings* (constriction in the throat, salivating, increased heart rate, excitement, longing, tension, withdrawal), or *images* (a nice red wine, an ice-cold beer, the smell of weed), or a *memory* of use. If you're feeling a craving right now in response to just thinking about alcohol/drugs, that's normal; don't fret. It just means it's even more important to continue reading, and it gives you a good chance right now to practice a helpful response to a craving.

What does a craving mean?

- **When your brain encounters a situation that it associates with prior drinking/drug use, the reward centers in your brain "light up" (become activated) and you experience a craving to drink/use drugs.** Reward centers are in the amygdala, a deep, primitive part of your brain that also motivates us to seek food, sex, and excitement.

- **A thought or picture or image of alcohol or a drug can elicit a craving, and your brain may actually start to release dopamine,** one of the primary brain "pleasure" chemicals that floods your system when you use drugs/alcohol.

- **You can't really control when a craving to drink or use drugs will happen.** You may learn to predict the possibility of a craving, but you can't stop it—it's similar to when you see food after not having eaten in a while and your mouth starts watering or your stomach starts grumbling. When you see a trigger for a drug or a drink, your brain will react and might release some dopamine even before you realize you have a craving.

- **A craving does not mean that you have to or should drink or use drugs!** A craving is simply a symptom of addiction. A craving may feel uncomfortable, but it will not hurt you in any way. A craving is simply alerting you that your brain reward and memory centers are activated. In fact, the only (non-medication) thing that will eventually stop cravings is to NOT use.

- Alcohol/drug cravings do NOT last forever! They are like waves in the ocean—they peak, they crest, and they subside. They usually go away in a short time. They will not hurt you. They will not kill you. They are just emotions. You can learn to tolerate and coexist with an uncomfortable emotion until it passes.

Tips to Cope with Cravings for Alcohol/Drugs

Use images to counter cravings:

- Picture bleach poured in the glass you usually drink from.
- Picture a dead spider floating at the bottom of a wine glass.
- Imagine a craving as a wave that comes and rocks the boat, but then passes you by.
- Picture an older woman sitting alone at a bar, drunk, eyes glazed.
- Picture a joint or pipe laced with fentanyl.
- Picture bleach in the syringe going into your veins.
- Picture your family grieving over you after an overdose.
- Imagine what you would do in this situation if there were no alcohol or drugs in the world.
- Imagine yourself in a pleasant place where you are peaceful, sober, and clear-headed.
- Imagine losing weight from no alcohol calories and zipping those jeans that used to be tight.
- Imagine being able to take a deep cleansing breath after not smoking or vaping for a while.
- Imagine what a non-drinker/user would do in this situation.

Cope with cravings through activity and distraction:

- If possible, get away from the situation that created the trigger.
- Find something fun to do that will get your mind off the craving to drink or use.
- Pray, read, eat, drink a non-alcoholic beverage, go to a movie, exercise, go to the gym, get involved with a hobby, take a walk.
- Journal.

Reach out to others:

- Talk/text about the craving with somebody who will be understanding.
- Ask someone you trust to help you when you are having a craving.
- Be assertive to protect yourself from cravings. Say "no" in advance to invitations/suggestions for activities that are high risk for you. For instance, say "no" to having alcohol in the house or "no" to having dinner at a bar; suggest a different activity to share.
- Be assertive if you're having a craving: "I'm sorry, I have to leave—I'm not feeling great/this is too hard for me. If you want to stay, that's fine. I'll call you later."

Use a relaxation technique:

▪ Do paced breathing (4-second inhale, 6-second exhale).

Use mindfulness:

▪ Observe the craving; do not try to control it. Do not act on it.

Talk yourself out of the craving:

▪ Remind yourself: No matter how bad, this craving will go away if I don't drink/use.
▪ **Remind yourself of the positive consequences and benefits of being abstinent.**
▪ Go through the list of reasons why you decided to stop drinking/using. Remind yourself about the bad parts of drinking/using.
▪ Say encouraging things to yourself that will make you feel good about not drinking/using.
▪ Tell yourself you can't always control when a craving comes, but you can just accept that "there's that craving again," and let it stay until it evaporates.

HANDOUT 6.4
Coping with Cravings: Sample Worksheet

Use images to counter cravings:

- Put pictures of my partner and kids on my phone screen to look at whenever I have a craving
- Imagine my son catching me sneaking a drink or a joint
- Imagine my kids seeing me passed out or being drunk or high and obnoxious
- Imagine my kids passed out from drinking if they learned it from me
- Imagine myself as an old lady sitting at a bar, nodding out
- Imagine what I would do right now if there were no alcohol or drugs in the world

Cope with cravings through activity and distraction:

- Ask my son to play basketball, or take a walk with me
- Go for a bike ride
- Get a cup of coffee/tea/seltzer with orange juice
- Go to the gym/pool/yoga studio
- Read a new novel I've been wanting to read
- Watch a funny movie

Reach out to others:

- Call or text my friend, sponsor, recovery coach, or therapist
- Call or tell or text my supportive spouse/partner that I'm having a craving to use
- Call or text a fellow group member

Use a relaxation technique:

- Try that new meditation app I downloaded
- Do paced breathing—take a deep breath, inhale 4 seconds, exhale 6 seconds
- Take a brisk walk or jog around the block to calm down and relax
- Dip my face in ice-cold water for 10 seconds while I hold my breath

Use mindfulness:

- Just observe and accept the craving and coexist with it until it goes away
- Observe the craving intensity and then note in an hour after not drinking or using that it went away
- Tell myself that this craving won't kill me and, while it's not comfortable, I can co-exist with it, observe how it feels, not act on it.

Talk yourself out of the craving:

- Tell myself it feels really strong now, but it will go away on its own if I don't drink/use and do something else instead
- Write what I love about being sober
- Challenge the thought "What's wrong with me? I'm hopeless, I'm a failure, still craving alcohol/drugs" with "That's shame I'm feeling. I have nothing to feel ashamed about. I realize I need to not drink or use and I'm working hard toward that goal."
- I'm doing okay; I've had several accomplishments this week coping with craving.

WORKSHEET 6.6
Coping with Cravings

Use images to counter cravings:

1. _____

2. _____

3. _____

4. _____

Cope with cravings through activity and distraction:

1. _____

2. _____

3. _____

4. _____

Reach out to others:

1. _____

2. _____

3. _____

4. _____

Use a relaxation technique:

1. _____

2. _____

3. _____

4. _____

Use mindfulness:

1. _____

2. _____

3. _____

4. _____

Talk yourself out of the craving:

1. _____

2. _____

3. _____

4. _____

Other:

1. _____

2. _____

Farewell to Members Leaving the Group (10 minutes)

Have members who are leaving identify the skills they think have been most important to the changes that they have made during therapy—that is, those skills they will continue to try to implement in order to maintain their progress. Remind group members that relapses most often occur in the types of situations they are now prepared to handle.

For women finishing the group, ask them how they feel about finishing the treatment program. Explore termination issues—fear, relief, loss. Discuss referrals for additional treatment if necessary. Discuss the possibility that group members may wish to stay in contact and provide support to one another.

Each group member who is finishing treatment should also be asked to go around the room and say something positive or constructive to each of her fellow group members. These statements could focus on positive changes or steps the leaving group member has seen each of the other women make during treatment, or ways in which the leaving group member feels she herself has learned or benefited from other women in the group. Other group members also should be encouraged to give some positive feedback to the woman who is finishing treatment. Women who are finishing treatment and the therapist may also want to say something to one another.

Anticipating High-Risk Situations This Week (5 minutes)

Rationale:

At the end of each session, we will spend a bit of time discussing any problem situations that each member thinks might come up around drinking or drug use this week. As you each progress through therapy, you will get better and better at anticipating and handling these. A "high-risk situation" is a situation in which you would find it very difficult not to drink. Today, I'd like us each to spend a few minutes together thinking about the upcoming week. [For each group member:] Are there any situations that you might encounter this week that would tempt you to drink or use drugs?

EXERCISE 6.5
High-Risk Situations and Executing High-Risk Situation Plans

Use Worksheet 6.7: High-Risk Situations, located in the Client Workbook:

Now let's each use Worksheet 6.7: High-Risk Situations to write in a high-risk situation for this upcoming week and brainstorm together about strategies/solutions you can use to cope with that high-risk situation in order to avoid drinking or using drugs in response to it. Are there any situations that you might encounter this week that would tempt you to drink or use drugs?

Elicit examples of upcoming high-risk situations from members and brainstorm together to generate plans for how to handle the situation for two or three group members. Write ideas about how to handle this situation on the High-Risk Situations worksheet. Refer to Session 1 in this guide for a copy of the worksheet or to the Client Workbook for a client version of the worksheet.

Assign Homework (5 minutes)

Here is a list of homework assignments for each group member to complete between today's session and the next. Remind the women how important it is to complete the homework.

1. Complete one self-monitoring card each day.
2. On the back of your self-monitoring cards, write down high-risk situations you encountered and how you handled them.
3. Read all the Session 6 material in your workbook and complete worksheets you didn't finish during the session.
4. Complete Worksheet 6.7: High-Risk Situations, located in the Client Workbook, and execute high-risk situation plans.

CHAPTER 12

Session 7: Affect and Mood Management

(Corresponds to Chapter 7 in the Client Workbook)

(1.5 hours)

Notes to the Therapist Before the Session

1. For rolling-admission groups (see Chapter 3), each new member should have an individual assessment (see Chapter 5) with the group facilitator prior to joining the group. At the end of the assessment session, for women joining the group at any session (i.e., Session 2–12) after Session 1, the therapist should spend an additional 30 minutes with each new group member to provide the Client Workbook and to review basic information covered in Session 1 that the client will need to know to proceed with all subsequent sessions. This includes coverage of use of the Client Workbook and group rules, as well as a brief review of core treatment elements, including self-monitoring, psychoeducation, high-risk situations, triggers, and behavior chains (see Session 2). That way, no matter what session the new member is entering, she will be able to do daily self-monitoring and understand the basics of high-risk situations, triggers, and behavior chains.

2. Each rolling-admission group session with a new member starts with a 5-minute round robin introduction of each group member, and 10 minutes of assessment feedback to the new member(s) (see Session 1 for detailed instructions and feedback sheets). Members in the group at different stages of recovery can provide support to the new client and share their own feedback from their first session. If a new member is lacking relevant information from previous sessions, she can review sessions in the Client Workbook or you can briefly describe the section, and/or abstinent members can be encouraged

to spend time with the new member after session to explain relevant prior material.

3. For each new member entering the group in Sessions 2 to 12, follow instructions at the beginning of each session regarding Introductions and Providing Assessment Feedback in Client's First Session.

4. If this is a client's first session, you must summarize data from the pretreatment assessment to fill in a Feedback Sheet (see Handout 1.10 in Client Workbook) for each client in the group in preparation for her first session.

5. Before the session begins, write the session agenda on a flipchart, whiteboard, or blackboard.

6. If you are doing the Optional Graphing Intervention, see instructions in Chapter 3 of this Therapist Guide.

7. All worksheets and handouts used in this treatment program appear in this Therapist Guide and in the corresponding Client Workbook; worksheets (and selected handouts) can also be accessed by searching for this book's title on the Oxford Academic platform, at academic. oup.com.

Session 7 Outline

All times are approximate and should be adjusted based on clinical need and whether group time needs to be devoted to new or departing members.

1. Pre-session sign-in and substance use check (15 minutes before session begins)

2. Introductions and agenda setting (5 minutes)

3. Check-in, review of self-monitoring and homework (20 minutes)

4. Cognitive and behavioral strategies to manage negative emotions, moods, and stress reactivity (50 minutes)

5. Farewell to members leaving the group (10 minutes)

6. Anticipating high-risk situations this week (10 minutes)

7. Assign homework (5 minutes)

1. Flipchart, whiteboard, or blackboard, felt-tip markers or chalk, eraser
2. Breathalyzer and tubes or saliva strips (optional)
3. Saliva drug tests for each group member (optional)
4. Seven self-monitoring cards for each group member (Note to therapist: Keep a stack of these to give group members at each session.)
5. OPTIONAL: Individualized graph for each woman
6. Handouts
   7.1: Types of Unhelpful Automatic Thoughts
   7.2: Challenging Unhelpful Automatic Thoughts: Example
   7.3: Automatic Thought Log—Anxiety: Example
   7.4: Automatic Thought Log—Depression: Example
   7.5: Strategies to De-stress and Manage Strong Negative Emotions
7. Worksheets
   7.1: Challenging or Letting Go of Unhelpful Automatic Thoughts
   7.2: Automatic Thought Log—Anxiety
   7.3: Automatic Thought Log—Depression
   7.4: High-Risk Situations [See Client Workbook Worksheet 7.4]

Pre-Session Sign-In and Substance Use Check (15 minutes pre-session)

If any member of the group appears to be high or intoxicated, you may want to assess her blood alcohol level (BAL) with a breathalyzer or saliva strip or use a saliva drug screen. Regardless of formal testing, though, if a group member is visibly high or intoxicated, review the treatment agreement with her and let her know that she will not be allowed to attend this session. Clients who miss a session will not receive a make-up session, but encourage them to read the handouts they missed for that session and complete the homework for the following week. You should assist the client in arranging alternate transportation home, review her abstinence plan, and remind her of her abstinence goal.

Introductions and Agenda Setting (5 minutes)

You will introduce new members joining the group this session, and provide an overview (i.e., set agenda) of what will be covered in the session and that the purpose of Session 7 is to: talk about strategies to cope with strong negative emotions associated with anxiety, depression, trauma, and shame. You can use these strategies along with some of the skills we learned in Session 5 and the information we covered in Session 6. Ask the group if there is anything pressing they would like to discuss today. Explain the absence of missing members without revealing protected health information.

Check-In, Review of Self-Monitoring and Homework (20 minutes)

Check-in follows a "round robin" format, in which drinking status and homework are emphasized. To introduce the round robin check-in:

We're going to go around the room using what we call a "round robin check-in" to get a brief version of how your week has been, focusing on your alcohol use, drug use, cravings, and triggers; how you coped with triggers and cravings; in hindsight what you might have done differently (with therapist and group input/ideas as well); homework you completed and what was helpful about it. We also will answer or clarify any questions or concerns about the homework material. Each group member will have a few minutes [depending on how many women there are in the group] to discuss with the group how your coping with alcohol/drug use triggers has been this week.

> **Therapist Note**
> *Try to pay particular attention to women's specific themes (e.g., right to self-care, empowerment) to link experiences to the specific theme: "One theme I've heard that's common among several of you is . . ."*

Go around the room and ask each group member how her week was (focusing on alcohol and/or drug use); listen while looking over her self-monitoring cards; and link what she is saying to her daily cards for alcohol/drug cravings, triggers, and use. Use information from this for specific topics in the rest of the session. Check in with each group member and discuss the progress of her abstinence plan. Update the plan if necessary. Also remember to ask each client at the end of her round robin time about what homework she was able to complete.

You should reinforce self-recording behavior, check for questions or problems, and help group members develop solutions for difficulties related to self-recording procedures. Ask members if they have any questions. Possible questions to anticipate include:

- **Question:** I thought about drinking the whole morning. Is that one urge or more than one?

THERAPIST: *You had the urge continually?*

CLIENT: Not every minute.

THERAPIST: *Well, each time you have a thought or an image about having a specific type of drink or a drink in a particular situation, that counts as a separate urge. Can you share some specific situations you thought about?*

- **Question:** Why are my urges so much higher than everyone else's? Why am I the only one still drinking?

THERAPIST: *It's natural that you would want to compare your drinking/ drug use and urges to those of the other group members. Although this can be an important motivator, it also is important to remember that everyone has her own unique path to abstinence. You're working on it, so be patient with yourself, and think of the changes you've already made! What does the group think about what _____ said?*

Therapist Note

After reviewing the daily monitoring cards, for outpatient settings you may wish to include the optional Graphing Intervention here.

Optional Graphing Intervention for Outpatient Treatment Settings

See the detailed instructions in Chapter 3 of this guide for how to use the graphs located in Session 2 of the Therapist Guide and the Client Workbook (Handout 2.1. Graph: Alcohol/Drug Use and Urges Sample and Worksheet 2.1. Graph: Alcohol/Drug Use and Urges). This intervention will allow each woman to track her progress by entering weekly data summarized from her daily monitoring cards: 1. Number of drinks; 2. Number of drugs used; 3. Number of urges/cravings; and 4. Average strength of urges/cravings.

Other Homework Review

Review all other homework clients did during the prior week. Reinforce clients for completing homework and discuss barriers experienced in completing the homework. Ask questions such as, *"What did you learn from the homework?"* or *"How can you use the homework to help you in the future?"*

Remember that as part of homework review, each week you need to review group members' recording of high-risk situations and how these were handled: *"Who wants to share how you handled one of your high-risk situations this week without drinking/using drugs?"* Elicit high-risk examples from two or three group members and get feedback from other members. Remember to have group members direct their comments to the other group members, and not just to you. Point out common types of high-risk situations among the group members and encourage women facing similar situations to share how they coped or ideas for coping. Selectively model and repeat empowering and motivational positive affirmations that group members give to one another: for example, *"We know this is hard, you're doing great." "Next time you'll be able to use a different strategy, hang in there."*

Also, ask about progress with doctor's appointments and blood tests. Due to time constraints, group members should discuss any concerns about their blood test or feedback with you after the group. Ask each client to bring in a copy of her lab results and give it to you. You can give feedback to the client during review of homework either that week or the week after.

Therapist Note

You should manage participation so that there is enough time to go around the room in a round robin fashion and give each group member a chance to speak. Keep in mind that 10 to 30 minutes total is allotted for check-in depending on how many women are in the group. If homework is not done, you should ask what made it difficult for the client to complete the homework. The importance of completing homework should be discussed, and a firm commitment for the future should be stressed in a nonjudgmental way.

Share the following with the group:

The time in the treatment group is only part of the process. The real change occurs when you practice changing your lives in the real world. The group will help you get ideas, stay motivated, keep you on track, and develop an understanding of the problem. But actually changing behavior takes place in your everyday life—at home, at work, with family, friends, and so on.

Therapist Note

The following are some tips for managing members' participation to maintain the temporal structure of the session: For habitually quiet members or those who appear upset or distressed, you should acknowledge them with empathic nonverbal behavior, but do not call on them to elicit participation right away, except during their turn in the round robin. Look for opportunities to invite limited participation of habitually quiet members to help them become comfortable sharing. Frequently ask the group for their feedback on particular group members' contributions, to set up the expectation that group members will be doing a lot of the work in the room. Everyone in the group learns by hearing the experiences and advice of others. Model and facilitate a tone of supportive, constructive, and compassionate feedback in the group. Don't be confrontational, but also don't condone or reassure a woman about her drinking/drug use or lack of work outside the group sessions. For instance, don't say, "It's okay. You had a really hard week; of course you drank a bit." Say instead, "You certainly had a hard week! In hindsight, what could you have done differently in response to trigger xxx?"

Group members who are having substantial difficulty with their abstinence plan or who appear to be at risk for an emergency should be asked discreetly to remain after group for an individual check-in with you.

Cognitive and Behavioral Strategies to Manage Negative Emotions, Moods, and Stress Reactivity (50 minutes)

Rationale:

In today's session, we will use some of the information we covered last week to teach you new ways to calm down and feel better. The goal is to train yourself to stop reacting to people and situations in ways that increase your negative emotions and decrease your self-confidence. The goal is to recognize when you're starting to become anxious or depressed, so that you can stop yourself from spiraling downward into uncontrolled anxiety or sadness.

Ask group members if any of this rings a bell, or bring in examples or ask volunteers to bring in examples from their own lives to illustrate the concepts.

Review and summarize with two or three volunteer clients the worksheets and homework from last week, to discuss which types of emotions and moods seem most problematic for them. Here are some suggested ways to frame these comments:

[Client A], it looks like anxiety is pretty tough for you, and you have a tendency to experience a spiraling effect in your anxiety. You start out being worried about something your boss said, and that spreads to work generally, paying the bills, the future, and so on, until you feel like it's all out of your control. Does this description sound like you? That's usually considered a type of "generalized anxiety."

[Client B], your pattern is a bit different. You might start out feeling a bit lonely, maybe in response to missing the kids, and that spirals into you feeling hopeless, beating yourself up about being a failure at marriage and being divorced, thoughts that you have hurt the kids by not staying married, and feeling quite depressed and overwhelmed.

The good news: You have more control over whether you feel anxious or sad in response to a situation than you think.

Just as there are triggers for drinking or using drugs, there are triggers for feeling anxious and sad. It's not always possible or desirable to avoid triggers for strong emotions, so today we will focus on changing your thoughts and responses to such triggers.

We will cover some general information to help you out here. First, we will cover "Challenging Negative Thoughts." Then, we will review some strategies to calm down and to manage strong negative emotions.

EXERCISE 7.1
Coping with Unhelpful Automatic Thoughts

In this exercise, clients will learn more about how their thinking can impact their emotions and mood and how they can cope with unhelpful thoughts. For this exercise, you will be using Handouts 7.1: Types of Unhelpful Automatic Thoughts and 7.2: Challenging Unhelpful Automatic Thoughts: Example and Worksheet 7.1: Challenging or Letting Go of Unhelpful Automatic Thoughts in the Client Workbook.

Thoughts run through our head constantly throughout the day; we talk to ourselves with these thoughts. They are called "automatic thoughts" because they happen very quickly, and are generated automatically in response to events/situations we encounter and are based on the habitual way we each think about and interpret the world around us. Automatic thoughts have great power over our mood and behavior, though we generally don't notice or recognize their effect. Some automatic thoughts are not helpful, and lead to anxiety and depression. These thoughts can be categorized into different general types; once they are categorized, we can label them and figure out how to handle them so that they do not automatically spark or worsen negative feelings such as anxiety and sadness.

*Events in our daily lives can trigger unhelpful automatic thoughts that then lead to negative feelings, which then lead to self-destructive behaviors. Our goal today is to help you learn to slow down the process of generating unhelpful automatic thoughts that go through your head and create or worsen negative emotions. We cannot always control events in our daily lives/environments, but we can generally control how we interpret and react to those events. We can learn to think about them in helpful, rather than destructive, ways. If you can learn to identify, challenge, and replace negative thoughts, you can start to learn to avoid anxious and depressed feelings and behaviors, or at least diminish their negative impact on you. Other tools to handle unhelpful automatic thoughts are also available, such as using a mindfulness approach to label, accept, coexist with, and let go of unhelpful thoughts, without their impacting our mood. A helpful thing to tell yourself is this: Thoughts are **not** facts! You can **choose** to go with negative thoughts or to **leave them behind!***

Let's look at Handout 7.1: Types of Unhelpful Automatic Thoughts—these will help us to figure out what category of thoughts we are having. [Review the different types of negative emotion thoughts, especially those types that seem most relevant to group members. Introduce the idea of classifying these thoughts into types; ask group members which types ring a bell.

Then we will look at the examples on Handout 7.2: Challenging Unhelpful Automatic Thoughts: Example to identify, challenge and replace or let go of unhelpful thoughts [Review the process of identifying, challenging, and replacing or letting go of unhelpful thoughts, while group members follow along.]

Then we will practice identifying, challenging, and replacing a negative thought or letting thoughts go, using Worksheet 7.1: Challenging or Letting Go of Unhelpful Automatic Thoughts.

Thoughts run through our head constantly throughout the day; we "talk to ourselves" with these thoughts. They are called "automatic thoughts" because they happen very quickly, and happen automatically in response to events/situations we encounter. Automatic thoughts can impact our mood and behavior, though we generally don't notice or recognize their effect. Here are some types of unhelpful automatic thoughts.

All-or-nothing thinking: This type of thinking ignores the possibility that some things are between all good and all bad. Example: *"I must always do a perfect job"* or *"I'm a failure."*

Catastrophizing: Exaggerates the importance and also the negative consequences of things. Example: *"Here I am, stuck in traffic. I'll be late to the meeting. My boss is probably ready to fire me."*

Over-generalization: Over-generalization happens when people see one bad experience as evidence of everything being bad. Example: *"My son got a C on that test. I don't help him enough with his schoolwork. I am a really bad mother." "I will always be depressed. This will never get better."*

Personalizing: Interpreting another person's behavior or a situation as implying something negative about you. *Example: "My neighbor passed me in the hallway at Back to School Night and didn't even look at me or say hello. I've always suspected that she doesn't like me, and now I know for sure."*

Mental filter: A negative mental filter keeps out positive thoughts and focuses on negative things. People see "the glass as half empty." Example: *"I look ugly—just look at my hair."*

Disqualifying the positive: This happens when a person believes that good things that happen somehow do not count. Example: *"I got a good grade on the test because it was so easy. Anyone could have gotten an A."*

Jumping to conclusions: People often jump to conclusions without having evidence to support their negative interpretations. *"My boss sent me that weird email because she wants me to quit."*

Mind reading: Assuming that you know what another person is thinking. Example: *"My husband looked at me funny. He hates this new outfit and is mad that I spent money on it."*

Depression filter: When people are depressed, they typically have thoughts that are quite negative, but this is because depression tends to distort the thinking process to result in an onslaught of negative self-talk. Example: *"I am really not where I should be at this stage of my life. At this rate, I have little hope for improving my future."*

"Should" statements: Some people set such high standards for themselves that they set themselves up for failure if they do not meet their standards of perfection. The key to catching this kind of thinking is the word *should.* Example: *"I should cook a full meal with a protein and vegetable every night for the family because that's what good mothers do."*

What if: This is a special type of anxiety thought that relates to worrying. People worry about their inability to do common everyday things (*"What if I run out of money this month and can't pay my rent?"*), or they worry about being or going crazy (*"What if I'm really nuts and I end up in a mental hospital?"*), or they worry about rare events (*"What if my doctor tells me I have cancer?"*), or they worry about having anxiety (*"What if I have another panic attack while I'm driving the car?"*).

Adapted in part from Burns (1989), *Feeling good: The new mood therapy.* William Morrow Books

Challenging Unhelpful Automatic Thoughts: Example

Sandra has been sober for 2 months now, thanks to hard work on her part. She is feeling particularly proud of herself this weekend. She managed to attend a wedding on Saturday and didn't have a slip even though there was an open bar. On Sunday morning, she is thinking that maybe she and her boyfriend, Abe, and his two kids will take a ride to the beach. But when he wakes up, he announces that he forgot to tell Sandra that he promised his kids that he would take them on a fishing boat that day. He tells her that she's welcome to come with them. Sandra feels herself getting upset. She thinks, *"I get nauseous on those boats, so I don't want to go. Now, I'll be stuck here all day alone, with nothing to do. My life is empty. I messed up my life and don't have my own kids. I'm such a loser—of course Abe doesn't want to spend the day with me."* In past similar situations she might have stayed quiet, cried when they left, and then stayed home watching TV and feeling sad.

Today, instead, she challenged and replaced, or let go of, her negative thoughts:

Negative Thought: (sadness)

Now I'll be stuck here all day alone, with nothing to do. My life is empty.

Challenge and Replace, or let thought go: (less sad)

Challenge and replace: *Wait a minute—I'm "over generalizing" - I'm not stuck. I can still go to the beach myself, or ask a friend. My life isn't empty.*

Let it go: *There's my mind going into the old "poor me" loop . . . it's not true and there's no point dwelling there.*

Negative Thought: (sadness)

I messed up my life and don't have my own kids.

Challenge and Replace, or let thought go: (neutral)

Challenge and replace: *This is "all or nothing thinking." What is a different way to think about this? I didn't want to have children with my ex-husband, and that was an excellent decision. When I met Abe it was too late for me to have a baby, and I'm lucky to have his kids in my life.*

Let it go: *Take a breath. Having that "I messed up my life" thought again – not useful, not even true.*

Negative Thought: (depression)

I'm such a loser. Of course Abe doesn't want to spend the day with me.

Challenge and Replace, or let thought go: (energized)

Challenge and replace*: That's my negative mental filter. Actually, Abe asked me to go with them, so that thought isn't true.*

Let it go*: It's okay to feel a little disappointed. But it's a beautiful day outside - I'll call my girlfriend to see if she wants to go to the beach.*

Challenging or Letting Go of Unhelpful Automatic Thoughts

Think about a situation where you felt depressed or anxious:

_____

_____

_____

Now, list the **negative thoughts** you had, along with the emotion that went with that thought.

Then write a thought(s) that challenges and replaces each negative thought.

1. **Negative thought** (emotion generated: _____)

_____

_____

Challenge and replace thought or let thought go (emotion generated: _____)

_____

_____

2. **Negative thought** (emotion generated: _____)

Challenge and replace thought or let thought go (emotion generated: _____)

_____

_____

3. **Negative thought** (emotion generated: _____)

Challenge and replace thought or let thought go (emotion generated: _____)

_____

_____

Clients can photocopy or download Worksheet 7.2: Automatic Thought Log—Anxiety and Worksheet 7.3: Automatic Thought Log—Depression to generate as many copies as they need for the week. Next week, you will review the logs and discuss what type of anxiety thought each is classified as according to the list of unhelpful thoughts and also will practice coping with the thoughts (challenge and replace, or mindfully let it go).

Automatic Thought Log—Anxiety: Example

Keep a log this week of thoughts that make you feel anxious. Rate each one from 0 to 10.

Date	Time	Situation	Thought	Anxiety Level (0–10)
8/1	4 am	Wake up, lying in bed	I'm so anxious. My heart is pounding. This feels awful. What if I can't get a full night's sleep all week?	9
8/2	6 am	Wake up	I didn't hear from my boyfriend last night – what if he was out and met someone else?	8
8/2	10 am	At work	I am overwhelmed. I'm an anxious mess. I can't possibly get everything done in time.	7
8/3	6 am	Wake up	What if I'm so anxious on the plane that I freak out?	7
8/4	4 pm	Getting ready to go out for dinner	I'm nervous about dinner - I might freeze and lose my train of thought again. I'll look so stupid and nerdy.	9
8/6	8 am	Driving to work	I acted like such an idiot yesterday—they will all know I don't know what I'm talking about. What if I lose my job?	8

WORKSHEET 7.2
Automatic Thought Log—Anxiety

Keep a log this week of thoughts that make you feel anxious. Rate each one from 0 to 10. We'll go over it next week.

Date	Time	Situation	Thought	Anxiety level (0–10)

HANDOUT 7.4
Automatic Thought Log—Depression: Example

Keep a log this week of thoughts that make you feel sad or depressed. Rate each one from 0 to 10. We'll go over it next week.

Date	Time	Situation	Thought	Depression Level (0–10)
9/6	4 am	Can't sleep, lay in bed	Oh my, I feel awful. So depressed. I don't want to go to work or do anything today. What's wrong with me?	9
9/6	6 am	Get out of bed	What's the point of showering? Too tired. I'll get the kids off to school and go back to sleep for a while. Can't face my meetings today. I don't contribute anyway.	9
9/6	3 pm	Driving to get the kids	Dragged myself through the morning routine. I feel awful. . What's the point? My life is so not where it was supposed to be at this age.	7
9/7	3:30 pm	Dinner prep time	I'm so tired. I can't take this feeling much longer. Ugh— have to choke down some food or will get a headache.	9
9/9	7 pm	Husband working late	Alone again. I've managed to alienate or isolate from everyone in my life who used to like me. Now no one calls or cares. Serves me right.	7

WORKSHEET 7.3
Automatic Thought Log—Depression

Keep a log this week of thoughts that make you feel sad or depressed. Rate each one from 0 to 10. We'll go over it next week.

Date	Time	Situation	Thought	Depression Level (0–10)

EXERCISE 7.2
Learning to Relax, De-stress, and Manage Strong Negative Emotion

In this exercise, you will practice strategies to handle anxiety, stress, and other strong negative emotions. For this exercise, you will be using Handout 7.5.

Let's discuss and summarize some skills to help you manage strong negative emotions. We will review Handout 7.5: Strategies to De-stress and Manage Strong Negative Emotions. This handout also includes a summary of how to handle anxiety and depression. We will discuss and circle the coping skills that seem most helpful and add your own. [You can also elicit group members' own strategies that have been helpful in managing negative emotions.]

Having a few simple, quick ways to relax can come in handy when you start to feel anxious or depressed. Here are some ways:

1. *Exercise: take a brisk walk, jog, or other exercise*
2. *When you feel tense, relaxation breathing can really help to relax you. It's quick and simple to learn.*

Paced Breathing for Relaxation

You may introduce paced breathing (also called "heart rate variability breathing") as follows:

Take a deep breath from your abdomen every 10 seconds, following these directions.
For the deep breath, put your palm on your belly and breathe in from your belly for 4 seconds, then out for 6 seconds. You don't need to hold your breath at any point. Keep your hand on your stomach to make sure it rises and falls when you breathe, so that you are breathing from your stomach, not your chest. The exhale has to be longer than the inhale—that's the most important thing. (It can be 5 seconds in, 7 seconds out, or 3 in and 6 out; whatever works best for you.) In between these deep belly breaths, breathe normally for 10 seconds. Then, repeat a 4-second-in, 6-second-out breath. Then, 10 seconds normal breathing. Then 4 seconds in, 6 seconds out, and so on. Do the paced breathing sequence once, or do it for 5 minutes, or 10 minutes.

Let's take a moment and practice here together. Put your hand on your belly. Take a deep belly breath in while you count silently to 4: 1 . . . 2 . . . 3 . . . 4 . . . Exhale while you count silently to 6: 1 . . . 2 . . . 3 . . . 4 . . . 5 . . . 6 . . . Breathe normally for 10 seconds: 1 . . . 2 . . . 3 . . . 4 . . . 5 . . . 6 . . . 7 . . . 8 . . . 9 . . . 10 . . . Deep belly breath in while you count to 4: 1 . . . 2 . . . 3 . . . 4 . . . Exhale while you count to 6: 1 . . . 2 . . . 3 . . . 4 . . . 5 . . . 6 . . . Breathe normally for 10 seconds: 1 . . . 2 . . . 3 . . . 4 . . . 5 . . . 6 . . . 7 . . . 8 . . . 9 . . . 10 . . .

Did anyone notice any difference in how you feel?

Another tip: We'll try it again, but now that you are used to breathing from your belly, keep doing that, but while you're doing the 4 in, 6 out, put a hand on each shoulder and gently push your shoulders down and back. Hold them there. That releases tension while you do the paced breathing. Here we go—remember to hold down and push back your shoulders. Take a deep belly breath in while you count silently to 4: 1 . . . 2 . . . 3 . . . 4 . . . Exhale while you count silently to 6: 1 . . . 2 . . . 3 . . . 4 . . . 5 . . . 6 . . . Breathe normally for 10 seconds: 1 . . . 2 . . . 3 . . . 4 . . . 5 . . . 6 . . . 7 . . . 8 . . . 9 . . . 10 . . . Deep belly breath in while you count to 4: 1 . . . 2 . . . 3 . . . 4 . . . Exhale while you count to 6: 1 . . . 2 . . . 3 . . . 4 . . . 5 . . . 6 . . . Breathe normally for 10 seconds: 1 . . . 2 . . . 3 . . . 4 . . . 5 . . . 6 . . . 7 . . . 8 . . . 9 . . . 10 . . .

How was that? [Elicit discussion/reactions in the group.]

For other ways to relax and de-stress, review Handout 7.5: Strategies to De-stress and Manage Strong Negative Emotions.

HANDOUT 7.5
Strategies to De-stress and Manage Strong Negative Emotions

❖ **Paced Breathing for relaxation:** "Paced breathing" (also called "heart rate variability" breathing) reduces stress/anxiety and resets your heart rate for more variability between heartbeats. More variability between your heartbeats is linked to relaxation, less depression, less anxiety, and less drinking.

- Stop, notice where you are tense, notice your shallow breathing.
- Breathe. Take a 4-second inhale from the belly—from the stomach, not the diaphragm (keep hand on stomach). Then do a 6-second exhale. **The exhale should always be longer than the inhale.**
- Breathe normally for 10 seconds. Then repeat 4-second belly inhale/6-second exhale.
- Do this paced breathing for 5 to 10 minutes.
- You may start to feel calmer and more clear-headed after even one breath.
- **Remember: The exhale has to be longer than the inhale—that is KEY.**
- During and after paced breathing, gently push your shoulders down and back.

❖ **"Diving reflex"**

- Hold your breath for 10 seconds while dunking your face in ice water (not below 50 degrees). Make sure your temples and the areas around your eyes are in the water.
- *Or* soak a washcloth in ice water and put it over your face.
- *Or* splash your face with icy water.
- This will instantly calm you down—it directs more blood/oxygen to your heart–brain circuit and lowers your heart rate.
- If it doesn't work at first, try it again.

❖ **Exercise**

- When acutely stressed, do a burst of fast, aerobic exercise for 15 minutes.

❖ **Ask yourself: Is this something I can control?**

- If it's not, go to acceptance and mindfulness strategies—let things go that you can't control. If you can control part of it, figure out what part you can control, and move on to problem-solving strategies.

❖ **Stop catastrophizing**

- Breathe as directed above and tell yourself you'll be fine.
- Ask yourself: Is this a catastrophe? What's the worst that will happen? What is plan B?

- ❖ **Talk yourself down**
  - ▒ Pick a mantra and repeat it. Examples:
    - ■ "Right here, right now."
    - ■ "Easy does it."
    - ■ "I know how to handle this."
    - ■ "I can't control this. Let it go."
    - ■ "Cool it. You're fine. You're safe."
    - ■ "Hold it—don't say or do anything you'll regret later."
- ❖ **Get up and do something** ("behavioral activation")
  - ▒ Lying around ruminating/thinking in loops over things that make you anxious or sad is not helpful. In fact, it makes things worse. Don't do it!
  - ▒ Get up, start your day, or take a walk, or get involved in an activity you used to find enjoyable or distracting.
- ❖ **Ask for help**
  - ▒ Talk to someone you trust.
- ❖ **Regain your calm and cool**
  - ▒ One of the destructive effects of strong emotion is physiological arousal, which causes mental confusion and has a bad effect on judgment. As long as you can regain your cool, you will be in control of the situation.
  - ▒ Human beings are animals with core brain structures designed to help us survive. When we were cave people facing a threat to our survival (like a lion or the threat of one), getting physiologically activated was adaptive to protect us by creating a fight-or-flight response. Now, when you stop short to avoid hitting a car, or face a danger walking home alone at night, this arousal system kicks into gear to help you survive.
  - ▒ However, because of our evolved brains and ability to imagine and remember, we can have many "false alarms." We may react to perceived threats of danger that are related to old emotional wounds or emotionally unsafe situations (neglect, criticism) that usually stem from childhood, betrayal, or a trauma. Situations that remind your brain of that past may stir up current physiological arousal and anxiety.
  - ▒ You can tell yourself to breathe deeply using paced breathing, and bring yourself back to the present. Tell yourself that this is a "false alarm"—there is no actual threat. Then, remind yourself that you are fine—it's just your body reacting to a perceived threat that isn't actually here.
- ❖ **Calm your physiology**
  - ▒ Take a hot bath, get a massage, or take a brisk walk or swim.

- ❖ Take a "time-out"
  - ▪ If you cannot immediately calm down, use a "time-out" to step away from the stressful situation for a few minutes and use any of the coping strategies described in this handout to give yourself time to get back in control of your anxiety or anger, and to avoid acting on your emotions or repeating past destructive behaviors.
- ❖ **Slow down** and assess the situation.
  - ▪ Identify, categorize, and challenge negative thoughts.
- ❖ **Talk to yourself with self-compassion and empowerment**
  - ▪ Remember, you are a good coper—you can cope with whatever comes your way; you just have to slow down and figure out the best way to proceed. Acting emotional will only make matters worse.
- ❖ **Acceptance: It's okay to feel sad or depressed. It's okay to feel anxious**
  - ▪ You may find that you cannot resolve the situation and you still feel sad. Remember that you can't fix everything. Let yourself feel sad—it's a natural feeling and will go away after a while.
  - ▪ Don't beat yourself up for feeling sad or depressed or anxious—you don't deserve it and that only makes things worse. Feeling sad or anxious won't kill you. Don't be scared by it.
  - ▪ You can't control whether or not you'll have anxiety or depression automatic thoughts. But you can control whether you let yourself get caught up in them, worry about them, obsess about them, and become even more anxious or depressed.
  - ▪ Anxiety and depression thoughts are like a snowball rolling down a hill. They pick up speed, size, and strength as they go, if you let yourself get caught up in them.
  - ▪ Instead, let the negative thought float in one ear, notice it, identify it and classify it, and then let it float out the other ear. It can't hurt you. You are safe. You're fine. Remember the mindfulness saying, "Thoughts are not facts." (Don't believe every thought that goes through your head.)
- ❖ **Congratulate yourself** for handling a difficult situation in a non-reactive way.
  - ▪ You behaved in a self-respectful way, and did not let others or your own emotion get the better of you.
  - ▪ You have also prevented yourself from spiraling downward into deeper anxiety or depression.

You may wrap up this part of the session as follows:

For homework, please read the handouts related to this topic. Please re-read all these handouts this week and complete any worksheets you didn't complete in session today. Also, keep a record of your unhelpful automatic thoughts this week on the worksheets provided (Worksheets 7.2 and 7.3) and we will discuss them next week. You can use the challenging unhelpful thoughts worksheet (Worksheet 7.1) this week as well if you want. There will be additional skills covered in Session 10 to manage anger and frustration.

Therapist Notes

1. *If individual group members have a diagnosable anxiety or mood disorder and need additional help, consider a referral for further evaluation or additional psychological care.*

2. *If at any point a client displays suicidal ideation, do a standard clinical suicide risk assessment and take appropriate steps to ensure the client's safety.*

3. *Be sure to communicate the following to clients who are considering medication to help with anxiety or depression:*
   Sometimes people experiencing anxiety and depression seek help from their physician and are prescribed medications to help them. You must be an educated consumer—be careful to avoid medications prescribed that are addictive, such as benzodiazepines (e.g., Valium, Xanax, Ativan, Klonopin), and often will create a new set of addiction problems for you. Withdrawal from a benzodiazepine, for instance, can be dangerous, even fatal, and weaning off regular use requires months of slowly reducing. We recommend asking your medical provider about the many non-addictive medications available to treat depression and anxiety. It's important to seek help for anxiety or depression from a qualified psychiatrist, preferably an addictions psychiatrist, if you feel you need additional help to get relief from anxiety and depression.

Farewell to Members Leaving the Group (10 minutes)

Have members who are leaving identify the skills they think have been most important to the changes that they have made during therapy, i.e., those skills they will continue to try to implement in order to maintain their progress. Remind group members that relapses most often occur in the types of situations they are now prepared to handle.

For women finishing the group, ask them how they feel about finishing the treatment program. Explore termination issues—fear, relief, loss. Discuss referrals for additional treatment if necessary. Discuss the possibility that group members may wish to stay in contact and provide support to one another.

Each group member who is finishing treatment should also be asked to go around the room and say something positive or constructive to each of her fellow group members. These statements could focus on positive changes or steps the leaving group member has seen each of the other women make during treatment, or ways in which the leaving group member feels she herself has learned or benefited from other women in the group. Other group members also should be encouraged to give some positive feedback to the woman who is finishing treatment. Women who are finishing treatment and the therapist may also want to say something to one another.

Anticipating High-Risk Situations This Week (10 minutes)

Rationale:

At the end of each session, we will spend a bit of time discussing any problem situations that each member thinks might come up around drinking or drug use this week. As you each progress through therapy, you will get better and better at anticipating and handling these. A "high-risk situation" is a situation in which you would find it very difficult not to drink. Today, I'd like us each to spend a few minutes together thinking about the upcoming week. [For each group member:] *Are there any situations that you might encounter this week that would tempt you to drink or use drugs?*

EXERCISE 7.3
High-Risk Situations and Executing High-Risk Situation Plans

Use Worksheet 7.4: High-Risk Situations, located in the Client Workbook:

Now let's each use Worksheet 7.4: High-Risk Situations to write in a high-risk situation for this upcoming week and brainstorm together about strategies/solutions you can use to cope with that high-risk situation in order to avoid drinking or using drugs in response to it. Are there any situations that you might encounter this week that would tempt you to drink or use drugs?

Elicit examples of upcoming high-risk situations from members and brainstorm together to generate plans for how to handle the situation for two or three group members. Write ideas about how to handle this situation on the High-Risk Situations worksheet. Refer to Session 1 in this guide for a copy of the worksheet or to the Client Workbook for a client version of the worksheet.

Assign Homework (5 minutes)

Here is a list of homework assignments for each group member to complete between today's session and the next. Remind the women how important it is to complete the homework.

1. Complete one self-monitoring card each day.
2. On the back of your self-monitoring cards, write down high-risk situations you encountered and how you handled them.
3. Read all the Session 7 material in your workbook and complete worksheets you didn't finish during the session.
4. During the week, keep an ongoing log of thoughts that make you feel anxious or depressed, using Worksheets 7.2: Automatic Thought Log—Anxiety and/or 7.3: Automatic Thought Log—Depression.
5. Using Worksheet 7.1: Challenging or Letting Go of Unhelpful Automatic Thoughts, practice challenging and replacing, or letting go of, anxiety or depression thoughts you notice and log.
6. Use relaxation skills twice this week; write down on the back of the self-monitoring card when you do.
7. Complete Worksheet 7.4: High-Risk Situations, located in the Client Workbook, and execute high-risk situation plans.

CHAPTER 13

Session 8: Connecting with Others, Dealing with Alcohol/Drug-Related Thoughts

(Corresponds to Chapter 8 in the Client Workbook)
(1.5 hours)

Notes to the Therapist Before the Session

1. For rolling-admission groups (see Chapter 3), each new member should have an individual assessment (see Chapter 5) with the group facilitator prior to joining the group. At the end of the assessment session, for women joining the group at any session (i.e., Session 2–12) after Session 1, the therapist should spend an additional 30 minutes with each new group member to provide the Client Workbook and to review basic information covered in Session 1 that the client will need to know to proceed with all subsequent sessions. This includes coverage of use of the Client Workbook and group rules, as well as a brief review of core treatment elements, including self-monitoring, psychoeducation, high-risk situations, triggers, and behavior chains (see Session 2). That way, no matter what session the new member is entering, she will be able to do daily self-monitoring and understand the basics of high-risk situations, triggers, and behavior chains.

2. Each rolling-admission group session with a new member starts with a 5-minute round robin introduction of each group member, and 10 minutes of assessment feedback to the new member(s) (see Session 1 for detailed instructions and feedback sheets). Members in the group at different stages of recovery can provide support to the new client and share their own feedback from their first session. If a new member is lacking relevant information from previous sessions,

she can review sessions in the Client Workbook or you can briefly describe the section, and/or abstinent members can be encouraged to spend time with the new member after session to explain relevant prior material.

3. For each new member entering the group in Sessions 2 to 12, follow instructions at the beginning of each session regarding Introductions and Providing Assessment Feedback in Client's First Session.

4. If this is a client's first session, you must summarize data from the pretreatment assessment to fill in a Feedback Sheet (see Handout 1.10 in Client Workbook) for each client in the group in preparation for her first session.

5. Before the session begins, write the session agenda on a flipchart, whiteboard, or blackboard.

6. If you are doing the Optional Graphing Intervention, see instructions in Chapter 3 of this Therapist Guide.

7. All worksheets and handouts used in this treatment program appear in this Therapist Guide and in the corresponding Client Workbook; worksheets (and selected handouts) can also be accessed by searching for this book's title on the Oxford Academic platform, at academic.oup.com.

Session 8 Outline

All times are approximate and should be adjusted based on clinical need and whether group time needs to be devoted to new or departing members.

1. Pre-session sign-in and substance use check (15 minutes before session begins)

2. Introductions and agenda setting (5 minutes)

3. Check-in, review of self-monitoring and homework (15 minutes)

4. Connecting with others: improving social support for abstinence (30 minutes)

5. Dealing with alcohol/drug-related thoughts (30 minutes)

6. Farewell to members leaving the group (10 minutes)

7. Anticipating high-risk situations this week (10 minutes)

8. Assign homework (5 minutes)

1. Flipchart, whiteboard, or blackboard, felt-tip markers or chalk, eraser
2. Breathalyzer and tubes or saliva strips (optional)
3. Saliva drug tests for each group member (optional)
4. Seven self-monitoring cards for each group member (Note to therapist: Keep a stack of these to give group members at each session.)
5. OPTIONAL: Individualized graph for each woman
6. Handouts
    8.1: Dealing with Thoughts About Alcohol and Drugs
    8.2: Dealing with Alcohol- or Drug-Related Thoughts: Sample
7. Worksheets
    8.1: I Want to Connect with People Who . . .
    8.2: Making Connections
    8.3: Dealing with Alcohol- or Drug-Related Thoughts
    8.4: High-Risk Situations [See Client Workbook Workssheet 8.4]

Pre-Session Sign-In and Substance Use Check (15 minutes pre-session)

If any member of the group appears to be high or intoxicated, you may want to assess her blood alcohol level (BAL) with a breathalyzer or saliva strip or use a saliva drug screen. Regardless of formal testing, though, if a group member is visibly high or intoxicated, review the treatment agreement with her and let her know that she will not be allowed to attend this session. Clients who miss a session will not receive a make-up session, but encourage them to read the handouts they missed for that session and complete the homework for the following week. You should assist the client in arranging alternate transportation home, review her abstinence plan, and remind her of her abstinence goal.

Introductions and Agenda Setting (5 minutes)

You will introduce new members joining the group this session, and provide an overview (i.e., set agenda) of what will be covered in the session. The purpose of Session 8 is to discuss what a supportive social network is, how to expand or use the network, and how to handle alcohol/drug-related thoughts without drinking/using. Ask the group if there is anything pressing they would like to discuss today in addition to the planned material. Explain the absence of missing members without revealing protected health information.

Check-In, Review of Self-Monitoring and Homework (15 minutes)

Check-in follows a "round robin" format, in which drinking status and homework are emphasized. To introduce the round robin check-in:

We're going to go around the room using what we call a "round robin check-in" to get a brief version of how your week has been, focusing on your alcohol use, drug use, cravings, and triggers; how you coped with triggers and cravings; in hindsight what you might have done differently (with therapist and group input/ideas as well); homework you completed and what was helpful about it. We also will answer or clarify any questions or concerns about the homework material. Each group member will have a few minutes [depending on how many women there are in the group] *to discuss with the group how your coping with alcohol/drug use triggers has been this week.*

> **Therapist Note**
> *Try to pay particular attention to women's specific themes (e.g., right to self-care, empowerment) to link experiences to the specific theme: "One theme I've heard that's common among several of you is . . ."*

Go around the room and ask each group member how her week was (focusing on alcohol and/or drug use); listen while looking over her self-monitoring cards; and link what she is saying to her daily cards for alcohol/drug cravings, triggers, and use. Use information from this for specific topics in the rest of the session. Check in with each group member and discuss the progress of her abstinence plan. Update the plan if necessary. Also remember to ask each client at the end of her round robin time about what homework she was able to complete.

You should reinforce self-recording behavior, check for questions or problems, and help group members develop solutions for difficulties related to self-recording procedures. Ask members if they have any questions. Possible questions to anticipate include:

▪ **Question:** I thought about drinking the whole morning. Is that one urge or more than one?

THERAPIST: *You had the urge continually?*

CLIENT: Not every minute.

THERAPIST: *Well, each time you have a thought or an image about having a specific type of drink or a drink in a particular situation, that counts as a separate urge. Can you share some specific situations you thought about?*

▪ **Question:** Why are my urges so much higher than everyone else's? Why am I the only one still drinking?

THERAPIST: *It's natural that you would want to compare your drinking/ drug use and urges to those of the other group members. Although this can be an important motivator, it also is important to re- member that everyone has her own unique path to abstinence. You're working on it, so be patient with yourself, and think of the changes you've already made! What does the group think about what _____ said?*

Therapist Note

After reviewing the daily monitoring cards, for outpatient settings you may wish to include the optional Graphing Intervention here.

Optional Graphing Intervention for Outpatient Treatment Settings

See the detailed instructions in Chapter 3 of this guide for how to use the graphs located in Session 2 of the Therapist Guide and in the Client Workbook (Handout 2.1. Graph: Alcohol/Drug Use and Urges Sample and Worksheet 2.1. Graph: Alcohol/Drug Use and Urges). This inter- vention will allow each woman to track her progress by entering weekly data summarized from her daily monitoring cards: 1. Number of drinks;

2. Number of drugs used; 3. Number of urges/cravings; and 4. Average strength of urges/cravings.

Other Homework Review

Review all other homework clients did during the prior week. Reinforce clients for completing homework and discuss barriers experienced in completing the homework. Ask questions such as, *"What did you learn from the homework?"* or *"How can you use the homework to help you in the future?"*

Remember that as part of homework review, each week you need to review group members' recording of high-risk situations and how these were handled: *"Who wants to share how you handled one of your high-risk situations this week without drinking/using drugs?"* Elicit high-risk examples from two or three group members and get feedback from other members. Remember to have group members direct their comments to the other group members, and not just to you. Point out common types of high-risk situations among the group members and encourage women facing similar situations to share how they coped or ideas for coping. Selectively model and repeat empowering and motivational positive affirmations that group members give to one another: for example, *"We know this is hard, you're doing great." "Next time you'll be able to use a different strategy, hang in there."*

Also, ask about progress with doctor's appointments and blood tests. Due to time constraints, group members should discuss any concerns about their blood test or feedback with you after the group. Ask each client to bring in a copy of her lab results and give it to you. You can give feedback to the client during review of homework either that week or the week after.

> Therapist Note
> *You should manage participation so that there is enough time to go around the room in a round robin fashion and give each group member a chance to speak. Keep in mind that 10 to 30 minutes total is allotted*

> *for check-in depending on how many women are in the group. If home-work is not done, you should ask what made it difficult for the client to complete the homework. The importance of completing homework should be discussed, and a firm commitment for the future should be stressed in a nonjudgmental way.*

Share the following with the group:

> *The time in the treatment group is only part of the process. The real change occurs when you practice changing your lives in the real world. The group will help you get ideas, stay motivated, keep you on track, and develop an understanding of the problem. But actually changing behavior takes place in your everyday life—at home, at work, with family, friends, and so on.*

Therapist Note

The following are some tips for managing members' participation to maintain the temporal structure of the session: For habitually quiet members or those who appear upset or distressed, you should acknowledge them with empathic nonverbal behavior, but do not call on them to elicit participation right away, except during their turn in the round robin. Look for opportunities to invite limited participation of habitually quiet members to help them become comfortable sharing. Frequently ask the group for their feedback on particular group members' contributions, to set up the expectation that group members will be doing a lot of the work in the room. Everyone in the group learns by hearing the experiences and advice of others. Model and facilitate a tone of supportive, constructive, and compassionate feedback in the group. Don't be confrontational, but also don't condone or reassure a woman about her drinking/drug use or lack of work outside the group sessions. For instance, don't say, "It's okay. You had a really hard week; of course you drank a bit." Say instead, "You certainly had a hard week! In hindsight, what could you have done differently in response to trigger xxx?"

Group members who are having substantial difficulty with their abstinence plan or who appear to be at risk for an emergency should be asked discreetly to remain after group for an individual check-in with you.

Connecting with Others: Improving Social Support for Abstinence (30 minutes)

Rationale:

In Session 3, we discussed how to manage heavy drinkers/drug users in your social support network as a way to help you become and stay abstinent. Today, we're going to discuss a related topic. It's very important to develop a stable personal support network of people whom you can enjoy, spend time with, turn to when you have troubles, and who appreciate you. Women in particular thrive better when they have a web of healthy connections with others. You have been learning to cope well, be autonomous, and take care of yourself—to be your own best friend. In addition to this, a supportive social network will enrich your life, provide you with opportunities for growth, offer warmth and happiness, and be there when you need a shoulder to lean on. Really, this next exercise is about self-worth: Do you truly believe that you deserve to surround yourself with supportive, respectful, and compassionate people? Do you believe that you have the right to choose not to spend time with or mental energy on people who are toxic for you, who do not treat you well, or who hurt you? This may be a new way to empower you, to think about choices you have the right to make.

EXERCISE 8.1
Social Support Network

In this exercise, clients will begin to evaluate their social networks and learn ways to enrich their networks with people who can provide them with positive support. For this exercise, you will be looking back at Worksheet 3.2: Your Social Network and Worksheet 8.1: I Want to Connect with People Who . . . and Worksheet 8.2: Making Connections.

> *Today, we will re-evaluate the social network support you have now versus when you began treatment. Then, we will discuss what you are looking for in members of your network. Third, we will discuss ways to reach out and develop a richer social network if that's what you feel you want to do. Part of self-care is providing yourself with a rich, healthy, connected network, and knowing when and how to reach out to people who want to help you. You don't need to do this alone.*

> *Let's update the social network graph (Worksheet 3.2: Your Social Network) you made in Session 3.*

Ask the group to look back at Worksheet 3.2. If a member is new to the group and has not yet participated in Session 3, you can give her a very short explanation of the worksheet and encourage a group member to show her a completed worksheet. Using this worksheet, ask group members to discuss any changes in their social networks since they last competed the worksheet. During this discussion, instruct group members to add any newly identified members to their own network, if relevant.

Therapist Note

As part of this discussion, ask group members to discuss how they think their social network may have changed over the past few weeks since they stopped or cut down their drinking or drug use. This discussion should include eliciting group members' feelings about whether they are content with their current support network for abstinence. Note that this exercise is designed to help each woman understand that she has the right to associate only with people who do not abuse her in any way, and who respect and nurture her. Then, ask group members to take out Worksheet 8.1: I Want to Connect with People Who . . . and take a moment to read it over and discuss it. Ask group members to list some other qualities that would be important to them in a person with whom they might establish or keep a connection. Encourage group members to list on their worksheets a few of the qualities they view as the most important. Encourage discussion among the group as the women complete the worksheet.

Continue this session as follows:

> *As we're looking over our social network worksheets, what are everyone's reactions to the way your own network currently appears or to any changes you've noticed in your network that have come about over the past several weeks while you've been reducing or stopping drinking/ drug use? Thinking about how important a healthy social network is in providing support for abstinence, do each of you feel satisfied with the current level of support you're receiving from your own networks? What about feeling connected with the individuals in your network, beyond their support for your abstinence? Let's look at Worksheet 8.1 to think about what sort of connections would feel best to you.*

WORKSHEET 8.1
I Want to Connect with People Who . . .

Circle any of these examples that resonate with you and then add your own.

I want to connect with people who.. .
   * I like and respect
    * I have fun with
     * I trust
      * I feel safe with
       * I care about
        * Care about me
         * Don't put me down
          * Respect my wishes
           * Are not always needy themselves
           * Know how to give and take
            * Have time for me
             * Understand addiction
              * Don't drink or use drugs
               * Don't hurt me—physically, verbally, or emotionally
                * Make me laugh and appreciate my humor
                 * Are not judgmental of me
                  * Are like-minded
                   * Make me feel heard and appreciated

* _____

* _____

* _____

* _____

* _____

When thinking about your social network, it might be helpful to ask yourself these questions:

*   Do I have people in my life who I feel I can count on when I need them?
*   Do I have people in my life who count on me?
*   Do I believe that others can help me?
*   How do I feel about others knowing that I have a problem and need them?

Next, you should ask group members to take out Worksheet 8.2: Making Connections. Point out that each group member can use any term she feels comfortable with—friend, significant other, social support person, etc. Then, have group members discuss what barriers they might experience in attempting to develop new friendships and how each individual group member can find ways to overcome these obstacles.

Let's look at Worksheet 8.2: Making Connections. We've talked about both the importance of social support networks and discovering the qualities we hope to find in the people who make up our own networks. Often women who are attempting to make changes to their social networks can encounter barriers or obstacles to seeking out new friendships and connections. Sometimes these obstacles can come from inside the woman herself, such as feeling anxious about meeting and striking up conversations with new people, or barriers can come from the woman's environment, for example having difficulty finding pockets of free time in her day to seek out new friendships. Let's work together on Worksheet 8.2 to see if you can be creative and come up with ways to add non-drinking/ using people to your social network. Then, for homework this week, finish Worksheets 8.1 and 8.2, and see if you can start to take steps to expand your social support network for abstinence.

Therapist Note

Do not allow the group to sit quietly while they each work on their own worksheets; rather, make this an open, interactive discussion of what group members are thinking about writing down. Group members can give each other feedback, support, and suggestions, and you can also chime in while each person also works on her Worksheet 8.2.

WORKSHEET 8.2
Making Connections

Some people are lucky enough to have great social networks "built in" to their families—supportive siblings, for example—or their neighborhoods. Others have to make more of an effort to develop a supportive social network. Let's brainstorm ways for you to connect with others to establish a strong, healthy social network. Social networks can consist of different types of "friends"—romantic partner/spouses, children, other relatives, female friends, male friends, AA/NA members, professional counselors, community-based networks, and so on. Let's brainstorm by category.

How can you . . .

. . . connect with female friends?

(volunteer organizations, yoga or other classes, Women for Sobriety, women-only AA meetings, reconnect with old friends)

_____

_____

_____

. . . connect with community-based networks?

(Smart Recovery Groups, AA, clubs, religious affiliations, special interest groups, meet-ups)

_____

_____

_____

. . . connect with family members?

_____

_____

_____

. . . connect in a healthy way with your romantic partner as part of your social support network?

_____

_____

_____

Rationale:

*I want to give you a slightly new way to think about drinking or drug use. Even though drinking alcohol or using drugs is a behavior (it's something you do), there are certain thoughts about alcohol and drugs that are more likely than others to lead to drinking or using. These thoughts usually run through our heads quickly and we often don't even notice them, or don't notice the effect they are having on our behavior. They are called "automatic thoughts" because they happen quickly. They are so familiar to us that we often don't notice them. They seem to happen automatically—they are "thought habits." We also term them as "unhelpful thoughts" if they lead to behaviors we are trying not to do. Today, we will learn about these types of thoughts that are related to drinking or drug use, learn to identify them when they happen, and learn how to deal with the thoughts about alcohol or drugs in a way that can help us develop more control over **cravings to drink or use and over drinking or using**. You probably have more control over determining the power of your thoughts than you realize!* Identifying and Challenging Thoughts That Lead to Drinking

Group members should follow along while you walk them through Handout 8.1: Dealing with Thoughts About Alcohol and Drugs. Elicit discussion as you go.

HANDOUT 8.1
Dealing with Thoughts About Alcohol and Drugs

Your thoughts lead to actions. You have control over what you do with your thoughts. Sometimes these thoughts happen so quickly that people believe they are acting without thinking. But if you could have an instant replay in slow motion, you could see how your thoughts lead to your actions.

Different types of thoughts can create urges that lead to drinking:

- **Thoughts or images directly about alcohol or drugs.** Some examples for alcohol are images of bars or of a favorite drink. Some examples for drugs are seeing a hash pipe or roach clip or being in the area where you used to purchase drugs. These thoughts directly trigger cravings.
- **"Permission" thoughts.** Some examples are "I can have just one, it won't be a problem." "I've been good; I can have one drink." "It's my birthday; I'll just take a couple of hits today." "No one will know."
- **"Expectation" thoughts.** Thoughts about the enjoyable effects of alcohol or drugs can trigger cravings: "A drink will calm my nerves." "A couple of pills will help me sleep." "A drink will help prevent nightmares." "I won't get through this party unless I get high." "A vodka will stop my mind from racing." These are called "expectation thoughts" about the short-term benefits of a drink or drug.
- **Negative thinking leading to negative feelings leading to drinking or drug use.** Unpleasant thoughts and emotions can lead to drinking or drug use. Some of these thoughts are about hopelessness or about negative self-worth and are sometimes called "F-it" thoughts. Negative thoughts may lead indirectly to drinking or drug use. They set up a chain of events that leads to drinking or using: "I can't believe I don't have a partner yet. I'll always be alone. I feel like crap; my life is pretty bleak. F-it. There's no reason for me to not get a little relief from a drink/drug right now."

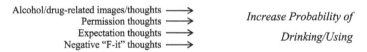

What to do?

- The first step is to **recognize the thoughts.** Be alert for these unhelpful thoughts.
- When you identify an unhelpful thought, challenge it and replace it with a more helpful thought.
- **Thoughts are not facts.** Don't take the thought seriously. Let it wander in one ear and out the other.

Remember the behavior chain? Focus on thinking all the way past using a drug or drinking!

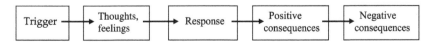

How to Break the Connection Between Thoughts and Drinking/Using

Rationale: Remind clients that their thoughts and what they do in a particular situation are linked. The goal of the next exercise is to deal with the thought so that it does not lead to drinking/using. This exercise will help group members learn how to modify their thoughts through cognitive restructuring. Emphasize that better control of their thoughts will make it easier for clients to control their drinking/using behavior. Ask for a volunteer to walk through Exercise 8.2 with you, while the other group members watch and offer suggestions and feedback and start to complete their own worksheet for themselves.

EXERCISE 8.2
Dealing with Alcohol- and Drug-Related Thoughts

Ask for a volunteer to offer examples of her alcohol- or drug-related thoughts and have the group help her to challenge them or use mindfulness techniques to accept, watch, and let them go. Work with the volunteer while you write her thoughts and the challenging thoughts on the flipchart/whiteboard. For this exercise, you will be using Handout 8.2: Dealing with Alcohol- or Drug-Related Thoughts: Sample and Worksheet 8.3: Dealing with Alcohol- or Drug-Related Thoughts.

> *You feel the "urge" to drink or use (i.e., you have a craving). Write down the positive thoughts you have about alcohol or the drug when you feel this urge. Then, think through the effects of drinking or using—getting drunk or high, neglecting your children, your partner or family getting very upset, looking awful, feeling ashamed, getting sick, and so on. Then, circle back to challenge the initial positive thoughts about alcohol or the drug and replace those thoughts with alternative ones about the reasons you don't want to drink or use. I'll write them down here.*

While you write the volunteer's thoughts on the flipchart, also have the group members write on their own worksheet personal examples of each type of thought they have experienced that has led to drinking or using. Then, give the group some time to complete their own worksheets, during which you should keep the discussion alive and interactive (i.e., don't just give 5 minutes of silent time to work on worksheets). Women should be sharing what they are writing and giving each other ideas and feedback. Then, ask for volunteers to share their own thoughts that have led to drinking or using. Generate more discussion.

HANDOUT 8.2
Dealing with Alcohol- or Drug-Related Thoughts: Sample

1. Direct, Positive Images or Thoughts About Alcohol or Drugs

That glass of wine looks inviting.

Everyone's so chill after a few hits of weed.

Challenge and Replace or LET IT GO

Looks can be deceiving. I'll end up drinking the whole bottle. It's not worth it.

Alcohol is a toxin. It is pickling my organs. And alcohol will actually make me thirstier. I'll have a seltzer and lime instead.

There's that thought again about the appeal of getting high. It's just a thought, not a fact; don't take it seriously. Doesn't mean I should actually take a hit. This thought won't kill me. I'll just let it hang around till it floats away.

2. Permission Thoughts

I've been really good. I can have one drink—no one will know.

Pat is away on a golf weekend. I'll take some "me time" with a joint outside on the deck; she'll never know.

Challenge and Replace or LET IT GO

Who am I kidding? I can't have just one drink. I'll end up drinking a bottle, eat a lot of junk food, probably start smoking weed too, and then want more tomorrow.

That's just a permission thought. There will always be an excuse. I'll just ignore that thought.

3. Expectation Thoughts

A few glasses of wine will help me get through the night with no nightmares.

I need to snort a line to stop feeling so lonely and depressed.

Challenge and Replace or LET IT GO

If I drink wine, I'll wake up in 4 hours. Better off taking my nightmare medication and chamomile tea.

Getting high is just a temporary fix, keeps me stuck. I'll try those stretches and breathing exercises to let
that thought ride out on an exhale.

4. Negative "F-it" Thoughts

I'm all alone here. No one cares about me. My life really sucks. F-it, I'll have some vodka.

I'm a failure—still struggling with drugs at my age. I'll never be well. F-it. Getting high will get rid of these feelings for a while.

Challenge and Replace or LET IT GO

Drinking just makes it worse. There's got to be a bright side here. I have my sister and brother. They care about me.

There's that "failure" thought again—my default automatic thought that makes me feel horrible. Just my brain doing its thing. I'm successful at work and I'm a great friend. I'm getting stronger every day; I don't deserve beating myself up like this. I'll force myself to go outside and take a walk, breathe the air, and focus on my legs moving. Good to get out of my head.

WORKSHEET 8.3
Dealing with Alcohol- or Drug-Related Thoughts

1. Direct, Positive Images or Thoughts About Alcohol or Drugs

_____

_____

Challenge and Replace or LET IT GO

_____

_____

_____

2. Permission Thoughts

_____

_____

Challenge and Replace or LET IT GO

_____

_____

3. Expectation Thoughts

_____

_____

Challenge and Replace or LET IT GO

_____

_____

_____

4. Negative "F-it" Thoughts

_____

_____

Challenge and Replace or LET IT GO

_____

_____

_____

Farewell to Members Leaving the Group (10 minutes)

Have members who are leaving identify the skills they think have been most important to the changes that they have made during therapy, i.e., those skills they will continue to try to implement in order to maintain their progress. Remind group members that relapses most often occur in the types of situations they are now prepared to handle.

For women finishing the group, ask them how they feel about finishing the treatment program. Explore termination issues—fear, relief, loss. Discuss referrals for additional treatment if necessary. Discuss the possibility that group members may wish to stay in contact and provide support to one another.

Each group member who is finishing treatment should also be asked to go around the room and say something positive or constructive to each of her fellow group members. These statements could focus on positive changes or steps the leaving group member has seen each of the other women make during treatment, or ways in which the leaving group member feels she herself has learned or benefited from other women in the group. Other group members also should be encouraged to give some positive feedback to the woman who is finishing treatment. Women who are finishing treatment and the therapist may also want to say something to one another.

Anticipating High-Risk Situations This Week (10 minutes)

Rationale:

At the end of each session, we will spend a bit of time discussing any problem situations that each member thinks might come up around drinking or drug use this week. As you each progress through therapy, you will get better and better at anticipating and handling these. A "high-risk situation" is a situation in which you would find it very difficult not to drink. Today, I'd like us each to spend a few minutes together thinking about the upcoming week. [For each group member:] Are there any situations that you might encounter this week that would tempt you to drink or use drugs?

EXERCISE 8.3
High-Risk Situations and Executing High-Risk Situation Plans

Use Worksheet 8.4: High-Risk Situations, located in the Client Workbook:

Now let's each use Worksheet 8.4: High-Risk Situations to write in a high-risk situation for this upcoming week and brainstorm together about strategies/solutions you can use to cope with that high-risk situation in order to avoid drinking or using drugs in response to it. Are there any situations that you might encounter this week that would tempt you to drink or use drugs?

Elicit examples of upcoming high-risk situations from members and brainstorm together to generate plans for how to handle the situation for two or three group members. Write ideas about how to handle this situation on the High-Risk Situations worksheet. See Session 1 in this guide for a copy of the Worksheet or to the Client Workbook (Worksheet 8.3 and 8.4).

Assign Homework (5 minutes)

Here is a list of homework assignments for each group member to complete between today's session and the next. Remind the women how important it is to complete the homework.

1. Complete one self-monitoring card each day.
2. On the back of your self-monitoring cards, write down high-risk situations you encountered and how you handled them.
3. Read all the Session 8 material in your workbook and complete worksheets you didn't finish during the session.
4. Take at least one action step toward the "new connections" ideas.
5. Complete Worksheet 8.4: High-Risk Situations, located in the Client Workbook, and execute high-risk situation plans.

CHAPTER 14

Session 9: Assertiveness Training and Drink/Drug refusal

(Corresponds to Chapter 9 in the Client Workbook)
(1.5 hours)

Notes to the Therapist Before the Session

1. For rolling-admission groups (see Chapter 3), each new member should have an individual assessment (see Chapter 5) with the group facilitator prior to joining the group. At the end of the assessment session, for women joining the group at any session (i.e., Session 2–12) after Session 1, the therapist should spend an additional 30 minutes with each new group member to provide the Client Workbook and to review basic information covered in Session 1 that the client will need to know to proceed with all subsequent sessions. This includes coverage of use of the Client Workbook and group rules, as well as a brief review of core treatment elements, including self-monitoring, psychoeducation, high-risk situations (see Session 1), triggers, and behavior chains. That way, no matter what session the new member is entering, she will be able to do daily self-monitoring and understand the basics of high-risk situations, triggers, and behavior chains.

2. Each rolling-admission group session with a new member starts with a 5-minute round robin introduction of each group member, and 10 minutes of assessment feedback to the new member(s) (see Session 1 for detailed instructions and feedback sheets). Members in the group at different stages of recovery can provide support to the new client and share their own feedback from their first session. If a new member is lacking relevant information from previous sessions, she can review sessions in the Client Workbook or you can briefly

describe the section, and/or abstinent members can be encouraged to spend time with the new member after session to explain relevant prior material.

3. For each new member entering the group in Sessions 2 to 12, follow instructions at the beginning of each session regarding Introductions and Providing Assessment Feedback in Client's First Session.

4. If this is a client's first session, you must summarize data from the pretreatment assessment to fill in a Feedback Sheet (see Handout 1.10 in Client Workbook) for each client in the group in preparation for her first session.

5. Before the session begins, write the session agenda on a flipchart, whiteboard, or blackboard.

6. If you are doing the Optional Graphing Intervention, see instructions in Chapter 3 of this Therapist Guide.

7. All worksheets and handouts used in this treatment program appear in this Therapist Guide and in the corresponding Client Workbook; worksheets (and selected handouts) can also be accessed by searching for this book's title on the Oxford Academic platform, at academic. oup.com.

Session 9 Outline

All times are approximate and should be adjusted based on clinical need and whether group time needs to be devoted to new or departing members.

1. Pre-session sign-in and substance use check (15 minutes before session begins)

2. Introductions and agenda setting (5 minutes)

3. Check-in, review of self-monitoring and homework (20 minutes)

4. Assertiveness training and effective communication (30 minutes)

5. Drink/drug refusal training (20 minutes)

6. Farewell to members leaving the group (10 minutes)

7. Anticipating high-risk situations this week (10 minutes)

8. Assign homework (5 minutes)

1. Flipchart, whiteboard, or blackboard, felt-tip markers or chalk, eraser
2. Breathalyzer and tubes or saliva strips (optional)
3. Saliva drug tests for each group member (optional)
4. Seven self-monitoring cards for each group member (Note to therapist: Keep a stack of these to give group members at each session.)
5. OPTIONAL: Individualized graph for each woman
6. Handouts
   9.1: Be Assertive, Not Passive or Aggressive
   9.2: Which Do You Do?
   9.3: Guidelines for Speaking Assertively and Communicating Effectively
   9.4: How to Refuse a Drink or Drug
7. Worksheets
   9.1: Assertiveness
   9.2: High-Risk Situations [See Client Workbook Worksheet 9.2]

Pre-Session Sign-In and Substance Use Check (15 minutes pre-session)

If any member of the group appears to be high or intoxicated, you may want to assess her blood alcohol level (BAL) with a breathalyzer or saliva strip or use a saliva drug screen. Regardless of formal testing, though, if a group member is visibly high or intoxicated, review the treatment agreement with her and let her know that she will not be allowed to attend this session. Clients who miss a session will not receive a make-up session, but encourage them to read the handouts they missed for that session and complete the homework for the following week. You should assist the client in arranging alternate transportation home, review her abstinence plan, and remind her of her abstinence goal.

Introductions and Agenda Setting (5 minutes)

You will introduce new members joining the group this session, and provide an overview (i.e., set agenda) of what will be covered in the session. The purpose of Session 9 is to talk about the right to ask for what you want and how to do that effectively. We also will apply assertiveness to how to refuse offers of alcohol or drugs in social situations. Ask the group if there is anything pressing they would like to discuss today in addition to the planned material. Explain the absence of missing members without revealing protected health information.

Check-In, Review of Self-Monitoring and Homework (20 minutes)

Check-in follows a "round robin" format, in which drinking status and homework are emphasized. To introduce the round robin check-in:

We're going to go around the room using what we call a "round robin check-in" to get a brief version of how your week has been, focusing on your alcohol use, drug use, cravings, and triggers; how you coped with triggers and cravings; in hindsight what you might have done differently (with therapist and group input/ideas as well); homework you completed and what was helpful about it. We also will answer or clarify any questions or concerns about the homework material. Each group member will have a few minutes [depending on how many women there are in the group] *to discuss with the group how your coping with alcohol/drug use triggers has been this week.*

> **Therapist Note**
> *Try to pay particular attention to women's specific themes (e.g., right to self-care, empowerment) to link experiences to the specific theme: "One theme I've heard that's common among several of you is . . ."*

Go around the room and ask each group member how her week was (focusing on alcohol and/or drug use); listen while looking over her self-monitoring cards; and link what she is saying to her daily cards for alcohol/drug cravings, triggers, and use. Use information from this for specific topics in the rest of the session. Check in with each group member and discuss the progress of her abstinence plan. Update the plan if necessary. Also remember to ask each client at the end of her round robin time about what homework she was able to complete.

You should reinforce self-recording behavior, check for questions or problems, and help group members develop solutions for difficulties related to self-recording procedures. Ask members if they have any questions. Possible questions to anticipate include:

- **Question:** I thought about drinking the whole morning. Is that one urge or more than one?

THERAPIST: *You had the urge continually?*

CLIENT: Not every minute.

THERAPIST: *Well, each time you have a thought or an image about having a specific type of drink or a drink in a particular situation, that counts as a separate urge. Can you share some specific situations you thought about?*

- **Question:** Why are my urges so much higher than everyone else's? Why am I the only one still drinking?

THERAPIST: *It's natural that you would want to compare your drinking/ drug use and urges to those of the other group members. Although this can be an important motivator, it also is important to remember that everyone has her own unique path to abstinence. You're working on it, so be patient with yourself, and think of the changes you've already made! What does the group think about what _____ said?*

> **Therapist Note**
> *After reviewing the daily monitoring cards, for outpatient settings you may wish to include the optional Graphing Intervention here.*

Optional Graphing Intervention for Outpatient Treatment Settings

See the detailed instructions in Chapter 3 of this guide for how to use the graphs located in Session 2 of the Therapist Guide and in the Client Workbook (Handout 2.1. Graph: Alcohol/Drug Use and Urges Sample and Worksheet 2.1. Graph: Alcohol/Drug Use and Urges). This intervention will allow each woman to track her progress by entering weekly data summarized from her daily monitoring cards: 1. Number of drinks; 2. Number of drugs used; 3. Number of urges/cravings; and 4. Average strength of urges/cravings.

Other Homework Review

Review all other homework clients did during the prior week. Reinforce clients for completing homework and discuss barriers experienced in completing the homework. Ask questions such as, *"What did you learn from the homework?"* or *"How can you use the homework to help you in the future?"*

Remember that as part of homework review, each week you need to review group members' recording of high-risk situations and how these were handled: *"Who wants to share how you handled one of your high-risk situations this week without drinking/using drugs?"* Elicit high-risk examples from two or three group members and get feedback from other members. Remember to have group members direct their comments to the other group members, and not just to you. Point out common types of high-risk situations among the group members and encourage women facing similar situations to share how they coped or ideas for coping. Selectively model and repeat empowering and motivational positive affirmations that group members give to one another: for example, *"We know this is hard, you're doing great." "Next time you'll be able to use a different strategy, hang in there."*

Also, ask about progress with doctor's appointments and blood tests. Due to time constraints, group members should discuss any concerns about their blood test or feedback with you after the group. Ask each client to bring in a copy of her lab results and give it to you. You can give feedback to the client during review of homework either that week or the week after.

Therapist Note

You should manage participation so that there is enough time to go around the room in a round robin fashion and give each group member a chance to speak. Keep in mind that 10 to 30 minutes total is allotted for check-in depending on how many women are in the group. If homework is not done, you should ask what made it difficult for the client to complete the homework. The importance of completing homework should be discussed, and a firm commitment for the future should be stressed in a nonjudgmental way.

Share the following with the group:

The time in the treatment group is only part of the process. The real change occurs when you practice changing your lives in the real world. The group will help you get ideas, stay motivated, keep you on track, and develop an understanding of the problem. But actually changing behavior takes place in your everyday life—at home, at work, with family, friends, and so on.

Therapist Note

The following are some tips for managing members' participation to maintain the temporal structure of the session: For habitually quiet members or those who appear upset or distressed, you should acknowledge them with empathic nonverbal behavior, but do not call on them to elicit participation right away, except during their turn in the round robin. Look for opportunities to invite limited participation of habitually quiet members to help them become comfortable sharing. Frequently ask the group for their feedback on particular group members' contributions, to set up the expectation that group members will be doing a lot of the work in the room. Everyone in the group learns by hearing the experiences and advice of others. Model and facilitate a tone of supportive, constructive, and compassionate feedback in the group. Don't be confrontational, but also don't condone or reassure a woman about her drinking/drug use or lack of work outside the group sessions. For instance, don't say, "It's okay. You had a really hard week; of course you drank a bit." Say instead, "You certainly had a hard week! In hindsight, what could you have done differently in response to trigger xxx?"

Group members who are having substantial difficulty with their abstinence plan or who appear to be at risk for an emergency should be asked discreetly to remain after group for an individual check-in with you.

Assertiveness Training and Effective Communication (30 minutes)

Rationale: People tend to have underlying beliefs about themselves and their world that they may not even be aware of; for women, a common underlying belief seems to be that they don't have the right to speak up for themselves about what they want, or even the right to have and voice a preference. On the other hand, some people have an oversized, entitled view of what they want and deserve, and that is not constructive either.

You may begin this part of the session as follows:

Today, we will talk about developing a different belief—that each person should be able to choose for herself how she will act in a given circumstance, after considering the rights of and respect for herself and of others.

Refer the group to Handout 9.1: Be Assertive, Not Passive or Aggressive, and ask the women to follow along while you provide the rationale. Elicit group discussion and share reactions and commonalities.

HANDOUT 9.1
Be Assertive, Not Passive or Aggressive

Conflict with others can lead to unpleasant emotions. For women especially, these emotions may lead to drinking or drug use. Many women have difficulty letting others know what they want and end up being too passive or too aggressive. Many women have not learned the basics of speaking assertively—the middle ground between passive and aggressive.

Passive behavior is usually based on a belief that you do not have the right to ask for what you want, or that you do not deserve to have what you want. A woman who chooses a passive response and puts the rights of others before hers most of the time may become "passive-aggressive," meaning that she is angry but does not outwardly express anger. Instead, for example, she may begin to gossip behind someone's back instead of figuring out how to communicate directly to get what she needs, or she may take on a project she doesn't think is fair and somehow sabotage the project by procrastinating. What often happens is that a person can be passive for a while, wanting to be a "good girl" or a "nice person," while building up resentment and then eventually exploding with **aggressive** behavior.

Women sometimes need to work on being more **assertive**. A feeling of self-confidence combined with self-compassion and with less focus on how other people might be thinking about you is a sign of increased "autonomy". Examples of thoughts that indicate assertiveness and a sense of autonomy are:

- "I can handle this. I can do this."
- "I deserve this. It's a reasonable request, and I'll ask politely."
- "This is my opinion, and I value it; so might others."

Greater autonomy usually helps us care less about what other people think us, and be less emotionally reactive to others. For instance, just because someone is angry at you does not mean you need to get angry back. Just because someone treats you with disrespect does not mean you should think less of yourself, or or get angry. Instead, you can take a step back to decide how you feel and what you think, take a deep breath, calm down, and decide how you wish to respond.

These situations can be difficult for women:

1. Frustration and anger situations
2. Making requests
3. Refusing requests
4. Giving/receiving criticism

These are situations in which assertiveness (not aggressiveness) may be helpful.

EXERCISE 9.1
Which Do You Do?

In this exercise, you will help clients to think about their own style of responding to situations and to try out a different way of interacting. For this exercise, you will be using Handouts 9.2: Which Do You Do? and 9.3: Guidelines for Speaking Assertively and Communicating Effectively, and Worksheet 9.1: Assertiveness.

Refer the group to Handout 9.2 and introduce this section as follows:

> *People generally choose one of three ways of responding to situations: They are passive, aggressive, or assertive. The gold standard is to be assertive, not too passive and not aggressive.*

Review Handout 9.2 and have group members volunteer to identify and discuss responses they typically use. Then, review Handout 9.3 and discuss. Then, using Worksheet 9.1, ask group members to volunteer examples of situations in which they think it would be helpful to be more assertive. You can help volunteers to come up with situations. Discussing the group's examples, work together to identify whether the volunteer is using a passive, aggressive, or assertive response in each situation. Then, do a role play as instructed here.

Instructions for Role-Play

Have a volunteer choose an example from her list and role-play an assertive response in that situation, using the information provided in Handout 9.3. First, you (the therapist) should role-play the client and model an assertive response to a situation the group member presents. Then, the volunteer should role-play an assertive response to a situation you present.

After the role-play, ask a volunteer to work through an example or two from Worksheet 9.1. Generate suggestions and discussions from the group during this exercise.

For homework, have each group member finish Worksheet 9.1 and identify two situations during the week in which she can practice using assertiveness skills. Have her write down these situations in real time on the back of her daily monitoring card.

Passive Behavior	Aggressive Behavior	Assertive Behavior
Self-denying ("Let him go first, even though I've been waiting longer.")	**Loses control of anger** ("These idiots had better give me what I want!")	**Feels good about self** ("I stayed in control, and I feel good about that!")
Inhibited ("I can't ask that—it may sound silly.")	**Chooses for others** ("Just do it my way and shut up.")	**Chooses for self** ("I am an adult; I can remain calm and ask for this.")
Hurt, anxious ("What if they don't like me?")	**Feels ashamed after losing control** ("I can never come back to this store.")	**Considers rights of self and others** ("I don't think I'm taking advantage. I have every right to ask this. It's fair to both of us.")
Allows others to choose for self	**Does not achieve desired goal** ("I stomped out and now I still can't return this stained shirt.")	**Usually achieves desired goal** ("Yes!")
Does not achieve desired goal ("Oh, well . . .")	**Does not consider others' rights** ("Just give me what I want!")	**Takes responsibility** ("It doesn't matter if life is unfair—I'm the one who loses if I don't try to take care of myself.")
Does not feel worthy of desired goal ("Oh, well . . .")	**Hurts others**	**Feels worthy of her own rights** ("I do deserve this!")
Resentment grows ("Why doesn't anybody see how hard I work?")	**Is unpopular**	**Thinks about how to word things** ("Let's see. Getting angry won't help. Take a deep breath and figure out how to say this in an effective way . . .")
Often results in explosive aggression ("I'VE HAD ENOUGH!")	**Feels out of control and stressed**	**Expressive**
Talks behind others' backs (Passive-aggressive)		**Feels calmer and in control**
Gossips (Passive-aggressive)		
Complains a lot (Passive-aggressive)		
Whines about unfair situation (Passive-aggressive)		
Does not take responsibility ("They are so unfair . . . no one sees that . . .")		
Feels helpless and depressed		
Does not command respect		

HANDOUT 9.3
Guidelines for Speaking Assertively and Communicating Effectively

Your Thoughts

- **Think about** how you want the situation to turn out.

- **Remind yourself** that getting angry will not achieve your desired goals and you will feel ashamed afterwards.

- **Remind yourself** that doing nothing also will not achieve your goals and you'll feel frustrated.

- **Try to think** about the situation from the other person's position.

- **Think about** how to word your request.

- **Talk** yourself through it.

Your Feelings

- **Label what you are feeling.**

- **Take a deep cleansing breath,** or use paced breathing (see Session 7) to focus and be calm.

- **When you feel really angry,** take a time-out.

Your Actions

- **Take action before you are too afraid to act, or so angry you can barely contain yourself.**

- **Look the other person in the eye.**

- **Speak up clearly and in a respectful but clear tone.** Don't apologize.

- **Use guidelines for good communication:**

- Be polite.

- Avoid blaming and sentences that begin with "you."

- Keep your voice tone pleasant.

Communicate Assertively:

1. Start with something nice, even if just a friendly greeting.

2. Calmly explain your position without blaming others.

(For example, instead of saying, *"Your store sold me a defective shirt with a stain on it and your return policy is ridiculous,"* say, *"Maybe you can help me—I bought this shirt here a few weeks ago and didn't notice until I went to wear it yesterday that it has a stain on it, which must have been there when I bought it. Unfortunately, it's past the return date according to the policy, but since I haven't worn it, I would like to exchange it for a similar shirt with no stain."*)

3. Start with an "I feel" statement whenever possible.

4. Explain what you are upset about.

5. Make a specific request for change.

No "grand slam" plays. Instead of storming out, be gently persistent.

(*"I see you're busy. May I speak with the manager, please?"*)

Here are some more tips for speaking assertively:

- Try to use statements that begin with "I feel." Remember to avoid statements that begin with "you." "You" statements make the other person feel attacked.

- Balance negative statements with positive ones, so the other person does not feel attacked.

- Recognize the other person's rights. If the person feels respected, he or she will be more likely to respect you.

- Request a specific change. Vague requests do not work because the other person is not clear about what you want.

- Clearly state what you want and why.

- Be firm in your answers to requests made by the other person.

- Speak loudly enough to be easily heard. Speak in a firm tone of voice.

- Don't hesitate a long time before speaking. Show you mean business.

- Look the other person in the eye. This tells the other person that you are confident.

Here are some tips for positive communication in general

1. Do's:

■ Be polite and treat everyone with respect—please, thank you, excuse me.

■ Remember to say what you appreciate about a situation or a person.

■ Choose the right time and place to bring up a problem.

■ Have a goal for every complaint.

■ Be brief and stick to one limited topic at a time.

■ Take responsibility for your role in things; stop the "blame game."

■ Self-soothe when you feel agitated before continuing the conversation.

■ Share your feelings: *"I feel* x *in situation* y *when you do/say* z.*"*

■ Try to understand and validate the other person's feelings and point of view.

■ Ask open-ended questions and listen carefully to the answers.

■ Monitor your nonverbals (make eye contact, keep voice tone calm, keep facial expression relaxed).

2. Don'ts:

■ Not listen. Focus on listening rather than on what you want to say next. Figure out what was intended, check if you understand, validate even if don't agree.

■ Interrupt. This is a conversation killer and makes communication ineffective.

■ Mind read. Don't assume you know what anyone else is thinking.

■ Insult. Insults, global criticism, and name calling—are all conversation killers. Stay away from "you always," "you never," "you are a . . .," or other insults.

■ Standoff/silent treatment routine. Take responsibility; don't blame and then ignore.

■ Devalue. Avoid saying things like, "That's ridiculous." Be respectful.

■ Ignore nonverbals: Don't raise you voice, scream, roll your eyes, stomp, sneer, ignore, slam doors.

WORKSHEET 9.1
Assertiveness

Think about your behavior in at least two situations in which assertive behavior could have been helpful. In the following columns, describe the situation, describe your response, and label your response as passive, aggressive, or assertive. We've given you an example in the first row to help you get started.

Situation	Your Response	Passive? Aggressive? Assertive?	Preferred Response?
Returning dress to store and cashier will not accept the return.	Lost temper, was nasty to cashier and stomped out without returning the dress.	Aggressive	Assertive and not nasty. Firmly but politely asked to speak with the store manager.

Rationale: Tell the group that the ability to refuse drinks or drugs is a special case of assertiveness, since ***one-third of clients with alcohol problems relapse as a direct result*** of social pressure from "friends" to drink, and as many as ***two-thirds of adults with drug problems say social pressure contributed to their relapse.*** Thus, the ability to refuse drinks or drugs is an important tool in each woman's toolbox of self-management skills and for the ability to make independent decisions. In the following exercise, the group will practice ways of refusing/turning down drinks or drugs to gain control in these tough situations.

Group members may say they don't need this skill: "Refusing drinks or drugs is not a problem for me." You can respond:

Not every skill we cover will be exactly relevant to everyone here; parts of this may nevertheless come in handy at some point for most people who struggle with alcohol/drug use.

Or you can say:

It may be that you drink or use alone most of the time and don't have a problem saying "no" to drinks or drugs when you're with others. This "How to Refuse a Drink or Drug" skill is also useful to use on yourself— when you have permission thoughts about drinking or using drugs, learn how to assertively say "no" to yourself. You can refuse silently, in your thoughts, or you can even say it out loud (surprisingly helpful).

EXERCISE 9.2
How to Refuse a Drink or Drug

In this exercise, you will teach clients how to refuse a drink or drug when offered to them. You will be using Handout 9.4: How to Refuse a Drink or Drug.

Review with the group and ask them to follow along with Handout 9.4. Generate discussion: Are there other ideas for saying "no"? Are there particularly difficult refusal situations that members have experienced? Here are some helpful examples.

1. You're at your brother's house on Christmas Day. It's a special occasion; you're with family and friends.

   He says—How about a beer?

   You say—No, thanks; I'd like a seltzer or soda, though.

2. A group of your friends stop by your house or approach you at a party and offer you a line of coke.

   They say—Hey, Jill, how about a line?

   You say—No, thanks; I'm not using any more.

   They say—Oh, come on, one line won't hurt you—what kind of friend are you?

   Or, *they say*—What's the matter, are you too good to get high with us?

   You say—No, just not using. I'm hungry, though—I'll go get something to eat.

HANDOUT 9.4
How to Refuse a Drink or Drug

One-third of problem drinkers have a slip because of pressure from others; as many as two-thirds of drug users say that social situations contributed to their relapse. **Refusing offers of alcohol or drugs is harder than most people think. It takes special skills to say "no" to alcohol or drugs.**

- Offers of alcohol and drugs come in many forms. Sometimes friends, coworkers, or family members put direct verbal pressure on you to join in with them. Sometimes they bring a drink or drug to you. Sometimes you may just be concerned about what others will think if you refuse. For instance, a waiter asking what you would like to drink can be difficult to negotiate without thinking, "If I don't order wine, my coworkers will think I'm an alcoholic."
- Some people are easier to refuse than others. Some will politely accept your first refusal. Others may get pushy.
- Refusing alcohol and drugs is an important assertiveness skill. The foundation of assertiveness skills is respect for your own needs, and less worry about what people might think of you.

These skills are difficult to use in a real situation. Social pressure is one of the most difficult problems that people face. You may know many people who drink or use drugs and expect you to use as well. They will have a difficult time accepting the change. Drinkers often worry, for instance, that if they say "no" to a glass of wine at dinner, everyone will "think I'm an alcoholic and can't drink."

- Think of different situations you may face. Develop some strategies for handling each.
- Practice how to use these skills.
- Practice at home—use the mirror.
- Practice in real situations when you feel ready.
- Challenge your beliefs about what others will think if you refuse a drink or drug.

How to Refuse Alcohol or Drugs

- **Keep in mind that individuals who strongly encourage you to drink or use are like** *pushers* **and must be discouraged, politely but firmly.**
- **Be firm without getting aggressive.** By using the following skills, you can refuse without coming on too strong:
  - **"No" or "no, thank you" should be the first thing you say.** Starting with "no" makes it tougher for the *pusher* to try to manipulate you.

- **Look the person in the eye when you speak.** Eye contact makes you come across as firm. Not looking the other person in the eye tells him or her that you are not sure about what you are saying.
- **Speak clearly and in a serious tone.** Your manner should say that you mean business.
- You have a right to say "no." You want to stay sober. It is your life that you are protecting. Do not feel guilty.
- You do NOT have to give reasons that you don't want to drink or use. It is **none of anyone's business.** You do NOT have to say, "I'm an alcoholic" or "I am a drug addict."

❖ **It is natural and common to worry about what others will think and let that guide your response. But challenge your thoughts about this, to protect your sobriety and self-care. Think instead:**
- "I don't need to give details."
- "Most people will not assume I'm not drinking because I'm an alcoholic."
- "Non-drinkers and non-drug users refuse all the time and don't think twice about it."
- "If they are pressuring me, it's their problem, not mine."
- "Is caring about what other people think more important than my sobriety?"

❖ **If you feel compelled to give a reason, be brief and general. What you say is totally up to you.** Examples:
- "No, thank you, I'm not drinking today."
- "No, thank you, I don't feel like getting high today."
- A better answer that is less likely to invite pressure down the road—and that doesn't say anything about your abstinence—might be "No, thank you, I've been focusing recently on healthy eating, drinking, and more exercise" or "No, thank you, alcohol doesn't really agree with me these days." Or best: "No, thank you. I've stopped using alcohol/drugs for health reasons."

❖ **Suggest alternatives.** If someone is offering you a drink, ask for something non-alcoholic. If someone is asking you to get into a risky situation, suggest something else that is not risky.

❖ **Change the subject to a new topic of conversation.** Get the *pusher* to think about something else.

❖ **Ask the person not to continue offering you alcohol or drugs.** Someone who is pushing you to drink or use is not respecting your rights. Politely ask him or her to stop: "Thanks for asking, but you don't need to keep asking. I'd rather stick to club soda with lemon."

❖ **Know your bottom line.** You are saying "no" out of respect for yourself. If the person keeps pushing, use your problem-solving skills. Remember, you can leave, get the person to leave, or get help from others.

In this exercise, you will guide clients to try out drink/drug refusal skills using a role-play exercise. Refer back to Handout 9.4: How to Refuse a Drink or Drug.

You may introduce this exercise as follows:

> *Remember our rule of thumb: Individuals who offer you drinks/drugs may mean well but must be discouraged politely and firmly. You have the right to step back (emotionally and physically) and think: "What do I want and need right now? How can I protect my sobriety? How can I say 'no, thank you' assertively, but not aggressively? Do I need to do anything else to protect my sobriety and take care of myself, even if others may be surprised or not like it or have to accommodate?" What concerns might you have about saying "no" to offers from peers, hosts, or waiters?*

Therapist Note

Help the women identify and challenge difficult thoughts that come up (e.g., "They'll think I'm an alcoholic." "They'll ask why I'm not using." "They'll tease me or criticize me." "I'm not ready to tell anyone that I'm trying to change." "They'll worry about me and why I'm not drinking." See Handout 9.4 for help with this.

Therapist Note

Many clients will say they don't need this skill, but it may become apparent in role-plays that they do need to, at a minimum, tune up their refusal skills. By role-playing first as the therapist, you can model effective refusal skills. Also, having the client first play the "pusher" will give you a clear idea of what sorts of social pressure the client is facing in her drink/drug refusal situations.

Ask for a volunteer to role-play assertive drink or drug refusal with you. Ask her to briefly describe a typical scene in which she had difficulty refusing a drink or drug or had been encouraged to drink or use (remember her completed functional analysis for examples), or a similar situation that is likely to come up in the future. **Note:** The role-play (including switching roles) should be brief—up to 5 minutes. **First, you (the therapist) should play the role of the client** and the volunteer group member can play the "pusher" so that you can model an appropriate assertive response to the situation. Then, debrief with some discussion, such as observations, thoughts, and feedback from group members; the volunteer's thoughts about your modeled response and whether she thinks that would be realistic for her to do; and concerns she might have. **Next, switch roles (with the same client). You play the pusher and have the volunteer refuse the drink or drug.** You and the group members can offer constructive feedback on the role-play. Then, ask for the volunteer to describe her reaction to the role-play and how it felt, and ask the group for reactions to the role-play. Have the group split up into pairs and role-play with one another, switching roles with each other (pusher/drinker or user). Finally, process the role-plays with a bit of group discussion.

Farewell to Members Leaving the Group (10 minutes)

Have members who are leaving identify the skills they think have been most important to the changes that they have made during therapy, i.e., those skills they will continue to try to implement in order to maintain their progress. Remind group members that relapses most often occur in the types of situations they are now prepared to handle.

For women finishing the group, ask them how they feel about finishing the treatment program. Explore termination issues—fear, relief, loss. Discuss referrals for additional treatment if necessary. Discuss the possibility that group members may wish to stay in contact and provide support to one another.

Each group member who is finishing treatment should also be asked to go around the room and say something positive or constructive to each of her fellow group members. These statements could focus on positive changes or steps the leaving group member has seen each of the other women make during treatment, or ways in which the leaving group member feels she herself has learned or benefited from other women in the group. Other group members also should be encouraged to give some positive feedback to the woman who is finishing treatment. Women who are finishing treatment and the therapist may also want to say something to one another.

Anticipating High-Risk Situations This Week (10 minutes)

Rationale:

At the end of each session, we will spend a bit of time discussing any problem situations that each member thinks might come up around drinking or drug use this week. As you each progress through therapy, you will get better and better at anticipating and handling these. A "high-risk situation" is a situation in which you would find it very difficult not to drink. Today, I'd like us each to spend a few minutes together thinking about the upcoming week. [For each group member:] *Are there any situations that you might encounter this week that would tempt you to drink or use drugs?*

EXERCISE 9.4
High-Risk Situations and Executing High-Risk Situation Plans

Use Worksheet 9.2: High-Risk Situations, located in the Client Workbook:

> *Now let's each use Worksheet 9.2: High-Risk Situations to write in a high-risk situation for this upcoming week and brainstorm together about strategies/solutions you can use to cope with that high-risk situation in order to avoid drinking or using drugs in response to it. Are there any situations that you might encounter this week that would tempt you to drink or use drugs?*

Elicit examples of upcoming high-risk situations from members and brainstorm together to generate plans for how to handle the situation for two or three group members. Write ideas about how to handle this situation on the High-Risk Situations worksheet. Refer to Session 1 in this guide for a copy of the worksheet or to the client workbook (Worksheet 9.2).

Assign Homework (5 minutes)

Here is a list of homework assignments for each group member to complete between today's session and the next. Remind the women how important it is to complete the homework.

1. Complete one self-monitoring card each day.
2. On the back of your self-monitoring cards, write down high-risk situations you encountered and how you handled them.
3. Read all the Session 9 material in your workbook and complete worksheets you didn't finish during the session.
4. Implement two strategies to connect with others to continue working on your social support network from last session.
5. Identify two situations during the week to use your assertiveness skills. Write on the back of your self-monitoring card what happened.
6. Practice drink/drug refusal skills in two situations, if relevant.
7. Complete Worksheet 9.2: High-Risk Situations, located in the Client Workbook, and execute high-risk situation plans.

CHAPTER 15

Session 10: Anger Management; Relapse Prevention I: Seemingly Irrelevant Decisions

(Corresponds to Chapter 10 in the Client Workbook)

(1.5 hours)

Notes to the Therapist Before the Session

1. For rolling-admission groups (see Chapter 3), each new member should have an individual assessment (see Chapter 5) with the group facilitator prior to joining the group. At the end of the assessment session, for women joining the group at any session (i.e., Session 2–12) after Session 1, the therapist should spend an additional 30 minutes with each new group member to provide the Client Workbook and to review basic information covered in Session 1 that the client will need to know to proceed with all subsequent sessions. This includes coverage of use of the Client Workbook and group rules, as well as a brief review of core treatment elements, including self-monitoring, psychoeducation, high-risk situations, triggers, and behavior chains (see Session 2). That way, no matter what session the new member is entering, she will be able to do daily self-monitoring and understand the basics of high-risk situations, triggers, and behavior chains.

2. Each rolling-admission group session with a new member starts with a 5-minute round robin introduction of each group member, and 10 minutes of assessment feedback to the new member(s) (see Session 1 for detailed instructions and feedback sheets). Members in the group at different stages of recovery can provide support to the new client and share their own feedback from their first session. If a new member is lacking relevant information from previous sessions,

she can review sessions in the Client Workbook or you can briefly describe the section, and/or abstinent members can be encouraged to spend time with the new member after session to explain relevant prior material.

3. For each new member entering the group in Sessions 2 to 12, follow instructions at the beginning of each session regarding Introductions and Providing Assessment Feedback in Client's First Session.

4. If this is a client's first session, you must summarize data from the pretreatment assessment to fill in a Feedback Sheet (see Handout 1.10 in Client Workbook) for each client in the group in preparation for her first session.

5. Before the session begins, write the session agenda on a flipchart, whiteboard, or blackboard.

6. If you are doing the Optional Graphing Intervention, see instructions in Chapter 3 of this Therapist Guide.

7. All worksheets and handouts used in this treatment program appear in this Therapist Guide and in the corresponding Client Workbook; worksheets (and selected handouts) can also be accessed by searching for this book's title on the Oxford Academic platform, at academic. oup.com.

Session 10 Outline

All times are approximate and should be adjusted based on clinical need and whether group time needs to be devoted to new or departing members.

1. Pre-session sign-in and substance use check (15 minutes before session begins)
2. Introductions and agenda setting (5 minutes)
3. Check-in, review of self-monitoring and homework (15 minutes)
4. Anger management (30 minutes)
5. Relapse prevention I: Seemingly irrelevant decisions (30 minutes)
6. Farewell to members leaving the group (10 minutes)
7. Anticipating high-risk situations this week (5 minutes)
8. Assign homework (5 minutes)

1. Flipchart, whiteboard, or blackboard, felt-tip markers or chalk, eraser
2. Breathalyzer and tubes or saliva strips (optional)
3. Saliva drug tests for each group member (optional)
4. Seven self-monitoring cards for each group member (Note to therapist: Keep a stack of these to give group members at each session.)
5. OPTIONAL: Individualized graph for each woman
6. Handouts
   10.1: Anger Behavior Chain—Example
   10.2: Time-Out
   10.3: Time-Out Do's and Don'ts
   10.4: Small Things Count
7. Worksheets
   10.1: Anger Behavior Chain
   10.2: Seemingly Irrelevant Decisions
   10.3: High-Risk Situations [See Client Workbook Worksheet 10.3]

Pre-Session Sign-In and Substance Use Check (15 minutes pre-session)

If any member of the group appears to be high or intoxicated, you may want to assess her blood alcohol level (BAL) with a breathalyzer or saliva strip or use a saliva drug screen. Regardless of formal testing, though, if a group member is visibly high or intoxicated, review the treatment agreement with her and let her know that she will not be allowed to attend this session. Clients who miss a session will not receive a make-up session, but encourage them to read the handouts they missed for that session and complete the homework for the following week. You should assist the client in arranging alternate transportation home, review her abstinence plan, and remind her of her abstinence goal.

Introductions and Agenda Setting (5 minutes)

You will introduce new members joining the group this session, and provide an overview (i.e., set agenda) of what will be covered in the session. The purpose of Session 10 is to discuss anger management and the first relapse prevention skill about making the least risky decisions each day to protect against alcohol/drug use. Ask the group if there is anything pressing they would like to discuss today in addition to the planned material. Explain the absence of missing members without revealing protected health information.

Check-In, Review of Self-Monitoring and Homework (15 minutes)

Check-in follows a "round robin" format, in which drinking status and homework are emphasized. To introduce the round robin check-in:

We're going to go around the room using what we call a "round robin check-in" to get a brief version of how your week has been, focusing on your alcohol use, drug use, cravings, and triggers; how you coped with triggers and cravings; in hindsight what you might have done differently (with therapist and group input/ideas as well); homework you completed and what was helpful about it. We also will answer or clarify any questions or concerns about the homework material. Each group member will have a few minutes [depending on how many women there are in the group] *to discuss with the group how your coping with alcohol/drug use triggers has been this week.*

> **Therapist Note**
> *Try to pay particular attention to women's specific themes (e.g., right to self-care, empowerment) to link experiences to the specific theme: "One theme I've heard that's common among several of you is . . ."*

Go around the room and ask each group member how her week was (focusing on alcohol and/or drug use); listen while looking over her self-monitoring cards; and link what she is saying to her daily cards for alcohol/drug cravings, triggers, and use. Use information from this for specific topics in the rest of the session. Check in with each group member and discuss the progress of her abstinence plan. Update the plan if necessary. Also remember to ask each client at the end of her round robin time about what homework she was able to complete.

You should reinforce self-recording behavior, check for questions or problems, and help group members develop solutions for difficulties related to self-recording procedures. Ask members if they have any questions. Possible questions to anticipate include:

- **Question:** I thought about drinking the whole morning. Is that one urge or more than one?

THERAPIST: *You had the urge continually?*

CLIENT: Not every minute.

THERAPIST: *Well, each time you have a thought or an image about having a specific type of drink or a drink in a particular situation, that counts as a separate urge. Can you share some specific situations you thought about?*

- **Question:** Why are my urges so much higher than everyone else's? Why am I the only one still drinking?

THERAPIST: *It's natural that you would want to compare your drinking/ drug use and urges to those of the other group members. Although this can be an important motivator, it also is important to remember that everyone has her own unique path to abstinence. You're working on it, so be patient with yourself, and think of the changes you've already made! What does the group think about what _____ said?*

Therapist Note
After reviewing the daily monitoring cards, for outpatient settings you may wish to include the optional Graphing Intervention here.

Optional Graphing Intervention for Outpatient Treatment Settings

See the detailed instructions in Chapter 3 of this guide for how to use the graphs located in Session 2 of the Therapist Guide and in the Client Workbook (Handout 2.1. Graph: Alcohol/Drug Use and Urges Sample and Worksheet 2.1. Graph: Alcohol/Drug Use and Urges). This intervention will allow each woman to track her progress by entering weekly data summarized from her daily monitoring cards: 1. Number of drinks; 2. Number of drugs used; 3. Number of urges/cravings; and 4. Average strength of urges/cravings.

Other Homework Review

Review all other homework clients did during the prior week. Reinforce clients for completing homework and discuss barriers experienced in completing the homework. Ask questions such as, *"What did you learn from the homework?"* or *"How can you use the homework to help you in the future?"*

Remember that as part of homework review, each week you need to review group members' recording of high-risk situations and how these were handled: *"Who wants to share how you handled one of your high-risk situations this week without drinking/using drugs?"* Elicit high-risk examples from two or three group members and get feedback from other members. Remember to have group members direct their comments to the other group members, and not just to you. Point out common types of high-risk situations among the group members and encourage women facing similar situations to share how they coped or ideas for coping. Selectively model and repeat empowering and motivational positive affirmations that group members give to one another: for example, *"We know this is hard, you're doing great." "Next time you'll be able to use a different strategy, hang in there."*

Also, ask about progress with doctor's appointments and blood tests. Due to time constraints, group members should discuss any concerns about their blood test or feedback with you after the group. Ask each client to bring in a copy of her lab results and give it to you. You can give feedback to the client during review of homework either that week or the week after.

Therapist Note

You should manage participation so that there is enough time to go around the room in a round robin fashion and give each group member a chance to speak. Keep in mind that 10 to 30 minutes total is allotted for check-in depending on how many women are in the group. If homework is not done, you should ask what made it difficult for the client to complete the homework. The importance of completing homework should be discussed, and a firm commitment for the future should be stressed in a nonjudgmental way.

Share the following with the group:

The time in the treatment group is only part of the process. The real change occurs when you practice changing your lives in the real world. The group will help you get ideas, stay motivated, keep you on track, and develop an understanding of the problem. But actually changing behavior takes place in your everyday life—at home, at work, with family, friends, and so on.

Therapist Note

The following are some tips for managing members' participation to maintain the temporal structure of the session: For habitually quiet members or those who appear upset or distressed, you should acknowledge them with empathic nonverbal behavior, but do not call on them to elicit participation right away, except during their turn in the round robin. Look for opportunities to invite limited participation of habitually quiet members to help them become comfortable sharing. Frequently ask the group for their feedback on particular group members' contributions, to set up the expectation that group members will be doing a lot of the work in the room. Everyone in the group learns by hearing the experiences and advice of others. Model and facilitate a tone of supportive, constructive, and compassionate feedback in the group. Don't be confrontational, but also don't condone or reassure a woman about her drinking/drug use or lack of work outside the group sessions. For instance, don't say, "It's okay. You had a really hard week; of course you drank a bit." Say instead, "You certainly had a hard week! In hindsight, what could you have done differently in response to trigger xxx?"

Group members who are having substantial difficulty with their abstinence plan or who appear to be at risk for an emergency should be asked discreetly to remain after group for an individual check-in with you.

Anger Management (30 minutes)

Rationale:

Today, we will take a closer look at "aggressive responses." Sometimes we find ourselves "flying off the handle"—losing our temper when someone or an unfair situation makes us mad. Some people tend to be "reactive" rather than "active." The problem with this is that anger takes a lot out of us, and leaves us feeling wound up and upset. Many people find that they drink or use to make themselves feel better after getting angry. Does this sound familiar to anyone? There is a better way to manage these types of situations.

EXERCISE 10.1
Anger Triggers

In this exercise, you will help group members learn more about effective and ineffective responses to frustrating situations and how thinking differently about a situation can help them respond more effectively. Use Handout 10.1: Anger Behavior Chain—Example and Worksheet 10.1: Anger Behavior Chain.

Imagine a bank manager getting annoyed at what she perceives to be an unfair decision during a staff meeting. Does she lose her temper and start to scream and cry? Does she yell and throw things? No, she remains "cool-headed" and is not reactive. She keeps her voice calm and explains in logical way why she disagrees with the decision. She still feels angry, of course, but she doesn't act on her anger in a destructive way.

Imagine a woman in front of you in line at a theater. She has lost her temper because she is told the movie she wants to see and arrived early to buy a ticket for is already sold out. She says loudly and in a nasty tone, "This is how you run this place? How was I supposed to know I need to buy tickets online?" Then, she stomps out of the theater yelling, "Never coming back here again!" Everyone in line just shakes their heads and goes on with their business. The woman did not get what she wanted and for the rest of the day she feels embarrassed and ashamed about her behavior in the theater.

Of these two scenarios, which way do you want to behave? Which way do you think commands more respect from others, more self-respect, and a higher chance that your opinion will be heard and valued? Losing your temper is usually not productive; you are unlikely to achieve what you want. Just because someone may try to provoke you into anger or into an argument doesn't mean you have to accept! We all feel annoyed at times, but expressing overt anger in words or actions usually makes us feel regretful and is not effective.

It is possible to handle almost anything that comes our way in a self-respecting, non-reactive manner, using problem-focused coping.

Let's take out Handout 10.1: Anger Behavior Chain—Example and Worksheet 10.1: Anger Behavior Chain. Take a minute to read over the example in Handout 10.1. As we read over this, let's discuss and list some of our own "anger triggers" that we encounter in our day-to-day lives. Would someone in the group be willing to work through an Anger Behavior Chain with me now, to discuss aloud a personal situation in the past that has served to trigger your own feelings of anger, and then come up with some possible strategies you could have used to calm yourself down? Say to the volunteer: *Let's complete an anger chain that you have noticed in the past, and then complete a chain for the same situation but swap in new, more helpful thoughts and responses. To help us come up with alternative thoughts and responses in our anger chains, you can look at Handout 7.5, Handout 10.2, and Handout 10.3.*

During the discussion, encourage group members should contribute to your helping the volunteer construct her anger behavior chain. While observing and contributing, group members also should be filling in one of their own anger behavior chains. You can also note that alcohol or drug use probably was one of their methods of coping with anger in the past, maybe even the primary method, and thus it is important for the group members to develop new ways of dealing with their triggers, challenging their angry thoughts, and learning alternative methods to calm down.

HANDOUT 10.1
Anger Behavior Chain—Example

Trigger	Unhelpful Thoughts/Feelings	Unhelpful Response	Positive Consequences	Negative Consequences
Received a child support check 1 week late and noticed that he deducted the cost of a toy he bought for our child	"What a jerk! He is not allowed to do that!" "Now he'll start deducting whatever he buys, and I won't have enough to pay the bills." "I need to give him a piece of my mind!" Anger, rage, burning up "I need a drink to calm down."	Call ex-husband, leave screaming message Have a few drinks	Momentarily relieved	Children say, "Mom, you're crazy!" Ex-husband plays taped message for the judge as evidence that kids are right. Feel ashamed and still angry Situation not resolved, and I drank

Trigger	More Helpful Thoughts/Feelings	More Helpful Response	Positive Consequences	Negative Consequences
Received a child support check 1 week late and noticed that he deducted the cost of a toy he bought for our child	"Of course I'm angry—he's an expert at pressing my buttons. I won't let myself suffer anger because of him." "I'll call my lawyer in the morning so this doesn't happen again, because it's not fair." "I feel sorry for him—doesn't he have anything better to think about in life than trying to push my buttons?" "I'm angry and I know that's normal, but I don't want to feel angry and don't want the anger to control me. I'm going to swim some laps."	Swim laps Take a walk Call lawyer	Feel less angry Proud of self—didn't lose control No screaming message taped to use against me Feel good that I didn't act crazy in response to ex Lawyer will help resolve situation.	Still feel a bit like screaming at him, frustrating

WORKSHEET 10.1

Anger Behavior Chain

Trigger	Unhelpful Thoughts/Feelings	Unhelpful Response	Positive Consequences	NegativeConsequences

Trigger	More Helpful Thoughts/Feelings	More Helpful Response	Positive Consequences	Negative Consequences

EXERCISE 10.2
Time-Out to Manage Strong Emotions

Use Handouts 10.2: Time-Out and 10.3: Time-Out Do's and Don'ts to introduce clients to time-out as a skill to manage and other strong emotions.

We've been talking about how to recognize anger triggers, how they contribute to alcohol and drug use, and some of the negative consequences of angry responses. In Session 9, we talked about how to be assertive, rather than passive or aggressive, in situations where you are upset or frustrated. Sometimes we feel so intensely angry that we find it difficult to think straight. Let's talk about that for a minute and then look at Handout 10.2 and Handout 10.3 together."

Ask the group if they have had this experience, and what has transpired when this happens. They may say they did or said something they regretted, got into an escalating argument with someone else, drank or used drugs, or just "lost it." Turn to Handout 10.2: Time-Out and Handout 10.3: Time Out Do's and Don'ts. Review the material on the handouts, asking group members for their reactions. Ask them what strategies they think would work best for them. Also, mention again that Handout 7.5: Strategies to De-stress and Manage Strong Negative Emotions is a great resource to learn emotion regulation and self-soothing techniques to reduce strong negative emotions.

"Time-out" means taking a break from a situation where you are getting angry or tense. You can also use this method if you are starting to feel anxious or depressed. Use a time-out to relax, think, cool down, and avoid being unreasonable, or even physical. Remember, it takes two people to make an argument. Just because someone else is angry doesn't mean you have to be. You are a separate person. It is your choice whether or not to engage in an argument; and it is your choice how to react to an unfair situation.

Below are the steps involved in taking a time-out:

Tell the other person that you are feeling tense and need some time to relax and think. It is important to communicate that you are not trying to avoid the problems and that you will be willing to talk about them later when you feel more relaxed and reasonable.

Get away from the person and the situation. It is best to leave the area altogether.

Do not drive a vehicle when really angry, or drink alcohol or use drugs during a time-out.

Calm yourself physically and mentally. Use a combination of physical and mental exercises that are non-aggressive. Concentrate on your breathing. Identify negative automatic thoughts that make you more upset. Practice challenging and replacing them with more helpful thoughts.

Give yourself time to relax and get control of yourself. When we get angry or anxious, our heart rate increases, blood pressure rises, blood sugar level rises, and certain other chemicals increase in our bodies. It takes time for our body to get back to normal. Give yourself at least 20 minutes, preferably 45 minutes to an hour, before returning to the situation.

Repeat, if necessary, the time-out procedure until there is no risk of getting out of control.

If you are with someone when you choose to take a time-out, it is important to tell the other person what you are going to do, where you are going (e.g., next room, to a friend's house), and when you will return (certain number of minutes/hours). *Example:* "I'm going to take a walk to cool off. I'll be back in about an hour."

Once you're calm, you can use your assertiveness skills to handle the upsetting situation.

Do's During a Time-Out

- *Do* practice positive self-talk:
  "As long as I keep my cool, I'm in control of myself."
  "I'm the only person who can make myself angry or calm myself down."
  "Time to relax and slow things down."
  "It's impossible to control other people and situations. The only thing I can control is myself and how I express my feelings."
  "It's nice to have other people's love and approval, but even without it, I can still accept and like myself."
- *Do* go for a walk, run, or swim to help work off some of the energy.
- *Do* think of constructive solutions to the problem.
- *Do* make use of your positive social connections—talk to a good friend.
- *Do* check in when you return home.
- *Do* let yourself have a good cry if you want to.
- *Do* let yourself feel sad if you need to. Then, let it go and allow yourself to feel hopeful.

Don'ts During a Time-Out

- *Don't* use alcohol or drugs. You will just create a new set of problems, and alcohol and some drugs increase hostility, anxiety, and depression. Using alcohol or drugs will make it impossible for you to gain self-control and self-respect.
- *Don't* talk with people who will feed your anger.
- *Don't* go to places where you have used alcohol or drugs in the past.
- *Don't* drive while angry. It is not only self-destructive but dangerous to others as well.
- *Don't* justify your anger or think about how wrong the other person is.
- *Don't* think about ways to control aspects of the situation you can't.
- *Don't* let yourself get sucked into anxious thoughts—let them come and go.
- *Don't* tell yourself you're crazy for feeling this way. You're not.

Rationale:

Many of the ordinary, mundane choices that we make every day seem to have nothing at all to do with drinking or drug use. However, although they may not involve making a direct choice to drink or use, they may move you, one small step at a time, closer to being confronted with that choice. Through a series of minor decisions, you may gradually work your way closer to the point at which drinking or drug use becomes very likely. These seemingly "minor" decisions that may, in fact, be risky and put you on the road to drinking or drug use are called "seemingly irrelevant decisions" because they don't seem to be relevant to alcohol or drug use—but they are.

EXERCISE 10.3
Seemingly Irrelevant Decisions

In this exercise, you will introduce the concept of seemingly irrelevant decisions to enhance client awareness of decisions that can increase their risk for drinking or using. For this exercise, you will be using Worksheet 10.2: Seemingly Irrelevant Decisions and Handout 10.4: Small Things Count.

Ask group members to take out Worksheet 10.2, which contains a story about a drinker explaining her most recent relapse.

WORKSHEET 10.2
Seemingly Irrelevant Decisions

Read the following story and underline the "seemingly irrelevant decisions" Georgia made that were high-risk and led to her slip.

Georgia decided to make a special dinner for herself and her husband, and she invited another couple to join them. She felt good about being abstinent from alcohol for the last 2 months and did not want to drink with dinner. However, she knew that the other couple liked wine and that red wine would go well with the menu she had planned. She also felt it would not be fair of her to deprive the others of alcohol. Therefore, she asked her husband to buy a couple of bottles of good red wine for the company. During the dinner, she felt comfortable not drinking. Her husband and their friends finished one bottle of wine and started the second. When Georgia was cleaning up in the kitchen after her friends had left, she looked at the almost full bottle of wine and decided it would feel good to have one glass and that she would then stop drinking. She had a glass of wine and then went on to have several more glasses, finishing the bottle.

Underline each one of the choice points where Georgia could have made a different decision that would have taken her away from a dangerous situation. What were Georgia's seemingly irrelevant decisions that resulted in her drinking?

List some safe choices versus risky choices in your own life:

Safe Choices	Risky Choices

After the group has identified several of these decisions, explain:

You have a greater chance to interrupt the chain of decisions that could lead to a relapse if you recognize what is happening early in a chain of events. This is important because it's much easier to stop the process early, before you wind up in a high-risk situation.

*You'll be able to recognize certain kinds of thoughts that can lead to making risky decisions, such as the thought that Georgia "**had to** serve wine with dinner" in the example. Thoughts like "I have to" go to a party, "have to" see a certain drinking friend, or "have to" drive by a particular place should be treated as warnings or "red flags." Other "red flag" thoughts often start with "It doesn't matter if I . . . " or "I can handle . . . "*

*Now that you've heard the story, you can see that Georgia made a series of decisions that led up to her final decision to take a drink of wine. (Did she really **have to** serve wine with dinner?) Georgia made a series of decisions, each of which contributed in some way to her finally taking the drink of wine.*

EXERCISE 10.4
Group Discussion of Seemingly Irrelevant Decisions and Risky Decision Situations

In this exercise, you will walk group members through Handout 10.4: Small Things Count. Then, you will guide discussion to help group members apply the concept of seemingly irrelevant decisions to their own situations.

HANDOUT 10.4
Small Things Count

Many of the ordinary choices you make every day seem to have nothing to do with drinking or drug use. Although these choices do not appear to be related to use, often you will find that small decisions lead to trigger situations. This is the "domino effect" of small decisions. One decision leads to another, which leads to another, and so on. A number of small "seemingly irrelevant decisions" may bring you closer to a high-risk situation.

Think about this story:

> *Sally needed a job and decided that, given her waitressing experience, she would look for a job in a restaurant. Clean and sober for 6 months, she felt confident that being around liquor in a restaurant would not make her want to drink. Sally got a job at a small BYOB seafood restaurant. After hours, the staff would often party by finishing off the bottles of wine left over by the patrons. One night Sally was waiting for a ride home after work with one of the other waitresses. Her favorite wine happened to be open on the counter. She thought, "It's been 6 months—I can handle one glass of wine." She drank a glass of wine, then two more glasses, then took a couple of hits off a joint that was being passed around.*

Sally made a series of decisions that led to her final decision to take a drink of wine and then smoke weed. For each one of the choices, Sally could have made a different decision that would have led her away from a risky situation. For instance, did she really **have** to stay after work when it was predictable that others would be drinking and smoking?

People often think of themselves as victims: "*Things just seemed to happen in such a way that I ended up in that situation and then I relapsed—I could not help it.*" They think things **happen to them** without realizing that many little decisions get them into trouble. That is because many of the decisions do not actually seem to involve drinking or using drugs. Each choice you make may take you just a little closer to drinking or using.

The best solution is to think about each choice you have to make. By thinking ahead through each possible option, you can look ahead for possible trouble. In the beginning, you may find thinking about every decision to be awkward. Eventually, you will find it easier to do.

To initiate and guide a discussion, ask group members:

Think about the most recent time you drank or used drugs when you were trying not to, and trace back the incident through the decision-making chain. What was the starting point— exposure to a trigger, or certain thoughts? Can you recognize the choice points where you chose to make a risky decision?

Then, ask group members to work together to come up with suggestions for low-risk options for the following seemingly irrelevant decisions situations in their own lives:

- Whether to keep alcohol or drugs in the house
- What sort of job to take
- What sort of social events to attend
- Whether to offer an ex-drinking/using friend a ride home
- Whether to go to a bar to see old drinking friends
- Where to go to get a snack
- Whether to tell a friend that you have quit drinking or using drugs or keep it a secret
- What route to take when driving (e.g., to go past or detour to avoid a favorite bar or place you used to buy drugs)

Farewell to Members Leaving the Group (10 minutes)

Have members who are leaving identify the skills they think have been most important to the changes that they have made during therapy, i.e., those skills they will continue to try to implement in order to maintain their progress. Remind group members that relapses most often occur in the types of situations they are now prepared to handle.

For women finishing the group, ask them how they feel about finishing the treatment program. Explore termination issues—fear, relief, loss. Discuss referrals for additional treatment if necessary. Discuss the possibility that group members may wish to stay in contact and provide support to one another.

Each group member who is finishing treatment should also be asked to go around the room and say something positive or constructive to each of her fellow group members. These statements could focus on positive changes or steps the leaving group member has seen each of the other women make during treatment, or ways in which the leaving group member feels she herself has learned or benefited from other women in the group. Other group members also should be encouraged to give some positive feedback to the woman who is finishing treatment. Women who are finishing treatment and the therapist may also want to say something to one another.

Anticipating High-Risk Situations This Week (5 minutes)

Rationale:

At the end of each session, we will spend a bit of time discussing any problem situations that each member thinks might come up around drinking or drug use this week. As you each progress through therapy, you will get better and better at anticipating and handling these. A "high-risk situation" is a situation in which you would find it very difficult not to drink. Today, I'd like us each to spend a few minutes together thinking about the upcoming week. [For each group member:] Are there any situations that you might encounter this week that would tempt you to drink or use drugs?

EXERCISE 10.5
High-Risk Situations and Executing High-Risk Situation Plans

Use Worksheet 10.3: High-Risk Situations, located in the Client Workbook:

Now let's each use Worksheet 10.3: High-Risk Situations to write in a high-risk situation for this upcoming week and brainstorm together about strategies/solutions you can use to cope with that high-risk situation in order to avoid drinking or using drugs in response to it. Are there any situations that you might encounter this week that would tempt you to drink or use drugs?

Elicit examples of upcoming high-risk situations from members and brainstorm together to generate plans for how to handle the situation for two or three group members. Write ideas about how to handle this situation on the High-Risk Situations worksheet. Refer to Session 1 in this guide for a copy of the worksheet or to the Client Workbook (Worksheet 10.3).

Here is a list of homework assignments for each group member to complete between today's session and the next. Remind the women how important it is to complete the homework.

1. Complete one self-monitoring card each day.
2. On the back of your self-monitoring cards, write down high-risk situations you encountered and how you handled them.
3. Read all the Session 10 material in your workbook and complete worksheets you didn't finish during the session.
4. Continue implementing strategies for connecting with others.
5. Use new skills on anger management this week if a situation arises; write on the back of a daily monitoring card what happened.
6. For seemingly irrelevant decisions homework, think about a decision you made recently or one you are about to make. The decision could involve any aspect of life, such as your job, recreational activities, friends, or family. Identify safe choices that might decrease your risk for relapse.
7. Complete Worksheet 10.3: High-Risk Situations, located in the Client Workbook Worksheet 10.3, and execute high-risk situation plans.

CHAPTER 16

Session 11: Problem-Solving

(Corresponds to Chapter 11 in the Client Workbook)
(1.5 hours)

Notes to the Therapist Before the Session

1. For rolling-admission groups (see Chapter 3), each new member should have an individual assessment (see Chapter 5) with the group facilitator prior to joining the group. At the end of the assessment session, for women joining the group at any session (i.e., Session 2–12) after Session 1, the therapist should spend an additional 30 minutes with each new group member to provide the Client Workbook and to review basic information covered in Session 1 that the client will need to know to proceed with all subsequent sessions. This includes coverage of use of the Client Workbook and group rules, as well as a brief review of core treatment elements, including self-monitoring, psychoeducation, high-risk situations, triggers, and behavior chains (see Session 2). That way, no matter what session the new member is entering, she will be able to do daily self-monitoring and understand the basics of high-risk situations, triggers, and behavior chains.

2. Each rolling-admission group session with a new member starts with a 5-minute round robin introduction of each group member, and 10 minutes of assessment feedback to the new member(s) (see Session 1 for detailed instructions and feedback sheets). Members in the group at different stages of recovery can provide support to the new client and share their own feedback from their first session. If a new member is lacking relevant information from previous sessions, she can review sessions in the Client Workbook or you can briefly

describe the section, and/or abstinent members can be encouraged to spend time with the new member after session to explain relevant prior material.

3. For each new member entering the group in Sessions 2 to 12, follow instructions at the beginning of each session regarding Introductions and Providing Assessment Feedback in Client's First Session.

4. If this is a client's first session, you must summarize data from the pretreatment assessment to fill in a Feedback Sheet (see Handout 1.10 in Client Workbook) for each client in the group in preparation for her first session.

5. Before the session begins, write the session agenda on a flipchart, whiteboard, or blackboard.

6. If you are doing the Optional Graphing Intervention, see instructions in Chapter 3 of this Therapist Guide.

7. All worksheets and handouts used in this treatment program appear in this Therapist Guide and in the corresponding Client Workbook; worksheets (and selected handouts) can also be accessed by searching for this book's title on the Oxford Academic platform, at academic.oup.com.

Session 11 Outline

All times are approximate and should be adjusted based on clinical need and whether group time needs to be devoted to new or departing members.

1. Pre-session sign-in and substance use check (15 minutes before session begins)
2. Introductions and agenda setting (5 minutes)
3. Check-in, review of self-monitoring and homework (15 minutes)
4. Problem-solving introduction and exercises (45 minutes)
5. Catch up on prior session material, review and consolidate what has been covered so far (10 minutes)
6. Farewell to members leaving the group (10 minutes)
7. Anticipating high-risk situations this week (10 minutes)
8. Assign homework (5 minutes)

1. Flipchart, whiteboard, or blackboard, felt-tip markers or chalk, eraser
2. Breathalyzer and tubes or saliva strips (optional)
3. Saliva drug tests for each group member (optional)
4. Seven self-monitoring cards for each group member (Note to therapist: Keep a stack of these to give group members at each session.)
5. OPTIONAL: Individualized graph for each woman
6. Handouts
   11.1: Problem-Solving Method
   11.2: Problem-Solving—Example
7. Worksheets
   11.1: Problem-Solving
   11.2: High-Risk Situations [See Client Workbook Worksheet 11.2]

Pre-Session Sign-In and Substance Use Check (15 minutes pre-session)

If any member of the group appears to be high or intoxicated, you may want to assess her blood alcohol level (BAL) with a breathalyzer or saliva strip or use a saliva drug screen. Regardless of formal testing, though, if a group member is visibly high or intoxicated, review the treatment agreement with her and let her know that she will not be allowed to attend this session. Clients who miss a session will not receive a make-up session, but encourage them to read the handouts they missed for that session and complete the homework for the following week. You should assist the client in arranging alternate transportation home, review her abstinence plan, and remind her of her abstinence goal.

Introductions and Agenda Setting (5 minutes)

You will introduce new members joining the group this session, and provide an overview (i.e., set agenda) of what will be covered in the session. The purpose of Session 11 is to cover a "general" coping skill (i.e., not directly to cope with alcohol or drug use) called problem-solving. Also ask the group if there is anything pressing they would like to discuss today. Explain the absence of missing members without revealing protected health information.

Check-In, Review of Self-Monitoring and Homework (15 minutes)

Check-in follows a "round robin" format, in which drinking status and homework are emphasized. To introduce the round robin check-in:

We're going to go around the room using what we call a "round robin check-in" to get a brief version of how your week has been, focusing on your alcohol use, drug use, cravings, and triggers; how you coped with triggers and cravings; in hindsight what you might have done differently (with therapist and group input/ideas as well); homework you completed and what was helpful about it. We also will answer or clarify any questions or concerns about the homework material. Each group member will have a few minutes [depending on how many women there are in the group] *to discuss with the group how your coping with alcohol/drug use triggers has been this week.*

> **Therapist Note**
> *Try to pay particular attention to women's specific themes (e.g., right to self-care, empowerment) to link experiences to the specific theme: "One theme I've heard that's common among several of you is . . ."*

Go around the room and ask each group member how her week was (focusing on alcohol and/or drug use); listen while looking over her self-monitoring cards; and link what she is saying to her daily cards for alcohol/drug cravings, triggers, and use. Use information from this for specific topics in the rest of the session. Check in with each group member and discuss the progress of her abstinence plan. Update the plan if necessary. Also remember to ask each client at the end of her round robin time about what homework she was able to complete.

You should reinforce self-recording behavior, check for questions or problems, and help group members develop solutions for difficulties related to self-recording procedures. Ask members if they have any questions. Possible questions to anticipate include:

- **Question:** I thought about drinking the whole morning. Is that one urge or more than one?

THERAPIST: *You had the urge continually?*

CLIENT: Not every minute.

THERAPIST: *Well, each time you have a thought or an image about having a specific type of drink or a drink in a particular situation, that counts as a separate urge. Can you share some specific situations you thought about?*

- **Question:** Why are my urges so much higher than everyone else's? Why am I the only one still drinking?

THERAPIST: *It's natural that you would want to compare your drinking/ drug use and urges to those of the other group members. Although this can be an important motivator, it also is important to remember that everyone has her own unique path to abstinence. You're working on it, so be patient with yourself, and think of the changes you've already made! What does the group think about what _____ said?*

> **Therapist Note**
> *After reviewing the daily monitoring cards, for outpatient settings you may wish to include the optional Graphing Intervention here.*

Optional Graphing Intervention for Outpatient Treatment Settings

See the detailed instructions in Chapter 3 of this guide for how to use the graphs located in Session 2 of the Therapist Guide and in the Client Workbook (Handout 2.1. Graph: Alcohol/Drug Use and Urges Sample and Worksheet 2.1. Graph: Alcohol/Drug Use and Urges). This intervention will allow each woman to track her progress by entering weekly data summarized from her daily monitoring cards: 1. Number of drinks; 2. Number of drugs used; 3. Number of urges/cravings; and 4. Average strength of urges/cravings.

Other Homework Review

Review all other homework clients did during the prior week. Reinforce clients for completing homework and discuss barriers experienced in completing the homework. Ask questions such as, *"What did you learn from the homework?"* or *"How can you use the homework to help you in the future?"*

Remember that as part of homework review, each week you need to review group members' recording of high-risk situations and how these were handled: *"Who wants to share how you handled one of your high-risk situations this week without drinking/using drugs?"* Elicit high-risk examples from two or three group members and get feedback from other members. Remember to have group members direct their comments to the other group members, and not just to you. Point out common types of high-risk situations among the group members and encourage women facing similar situations to share how they coped or ideas for coping. Selectively model and repeat empowering and motivational positive affirmations that group members give to one another: for example, *"We know this is hard, you're doing great." "Next time you'll be able to use a different strategy, hang in there."*

Also, ask about progress with doctor's appointments and blood tests. Due to time constraints, group members should discuss any concerns about their blood test or feedback with you after the group. Ask each client to bring in a copy of her lab results and give it to you. You can give feedback to the client during review of homework either that week or the week after.

Therapist Note

You should manage participation so that there is enough time to go around the room in a round robin fashion and give each group member a chance to speak. Keep in mind that 10 to 30 minutes total is allotted for check-in depending on how many women are in the group. If homework is not done, you should ask what made it difficult for the client to complete the homework. The importance of completing homework should be discussed, and a firm commitment for the future should be stressed in a nonjudgmental way.

Share the following with the group:

The time in the treatment group is only part of the process. The real change occurs when you practice changing your lives in the real world. The group will help you get ideas, stay motivated, keep you on track, and develop an understanding of the problem. But actually changing behavior takes place in your everyday life—at home, at work, with family, friends, and so on.

Therapist Note

The following are some tips for managing members' participation to maintain the temporal structure of the session: For habitually quiet members or those who appear upset or distressed, you should acknowledge them with empathic nonverbal behavior, but do not call on them to elicit participation right away, except during their turn in the round robin. Look for opportunities to invite limited participation of habitually quiet members to help them become comfortable sharing. Frequently ask the group for their feedback on particular group members' contributions, to set up the expectation that group members will be doing a lot of the work in the room. Everyone in the group learns by hearing the experiences and advice of others. Model and facilitate a tone of supportive, constructive, and compassionate feedback in the group. Don't be confrontational, but also don't condone or reassure a woman about her drinking/drug use or lack of work outside the group sessions. For instance, don't say, "It's okay. You had a really hard week; of course you drank a bit." Say instead, "You certainly had a hard week! In hindsight, what could you have done differently in response to trigger xxx?"

Group members who are having substantial difficulty with their abstinence plan or who appear to be at risk for an emergency should be asked discreetly to remain after group for an individual check-in with you.

Problem-Solving Introduction and Exercises (45 minutes)

Rationale:

In this session, we will focus on using problem-solving as a general coping skill. Sometimes people lack appropriate, positive coping skills to deal with difficult problems or situations in their lives and, hence, they develop a habit of drinking or using drugs to "cope" with those problems. Substance use is not an effective coping strategy to make problems go away in the long run; it is an avoidance coping strategy that makes you not care about the problem in the short term. In the long term, drinking or using drugs usually makes the problem worse and creates a new problem—the addiction. You can learn more effective coping skills to apply to problems and challenging situations in your daily life instead of drinking or using drugs to cope.

Briefly describe two types of coping strategies that people tend to use:

Emotion-focused coping *is when you get caught up in and focus on negative emotions (anger, sadness, frustration) associated with a life problem, and then often feel the need to escape from these feelings (i.e., by drinking or using, so as not to care about the problem in the short term). I am not saying that you should ignore your emotions—they are often a signal that there is a problem for you to solve—but reacting only with your emotions often leads to bad outcomes. Do not be afraid of your emotions. Notice them, allow them to float, and label them ("There's that sadness, anger, etc."). You can also use strategies in Handout 7.5: Strategies to De-stress and Manage Strong Negative Emotions to regulate them so they are less uncomfortable.*

The objective of this session is to help you learn to use your full brain, not just the emotional parts, to solve problems. This different coping strategy is called **problem-focused coping**. *You can notice and tolerate difficult emotions but manage your emotions so that you can deal with the problem effectively in a relatively clear-headed way. If you feel overwhelmed by emotion in response to a particular problem, you will need to calm yourself down before you attempt to do the problem-solving exercise. You can use some of the time-out strategies we talked about in Session 10 and emotion regulation in Session 7, such as paced breathing, burst of exercise, and challenging negative thoughts.*

Learning to be a good "coper" will increase your self-confidence, feelings of autonomy, and ability to be less reactive to people around you. The world will feel like a safer place, since you will be in a better position to protect yourself when things "go wrong." You can think, "Wait a minute here! This is not a catastrophe; don't panic. I can figure this out. There must be some options that I can try for the parts of this that I can control, and for the parts I can't control, I will need to figure out a way to let some of it go. I can do this. I've dealt with worse. Step away from these strong feelings, take a deep breath, and think through your options."

EXERCISE 11.1
Problem-Solving

In this exercise, you will introduce problem-solving as a skill. It is important that you empha-size problem-solving *techniques*, rather than only trying to solve a specific problem, in order to increase generalization. For this exercise, you will be using Handouts 11.1: Problem-Solving Method and 11.2: Problem-Solving—Example and Worksheet 11.1: Problem-Solving.

Review Handout 11.1: Problem-Solving Method, and discuss the general outline of problem-solving procedures. Explain that problem-solving consists of seven steps (have group members follow along on the handout).

Explain to the group members that problem-solving techniques can be applied to almost any problematic situation in their lives. Then, have group members go over Handout 11.2: Problem-Solving—Example and discuss what they think the optimal solution for Susan might be. Then, model the problem-solving method by working with a group volunteer to complete Worksheet 11.1.

Ask for a volunteer to offer a problem to demonstrate use of these techniques, while group members help out. Together with the volunteer, choose a problem that has come up over the sessions. The sample problem should be not impossibly difficult to solve, but not terribly easy to solve either. (We want this problem-solving exercise to be a good teaching tool for the group.) Follow the steps below:

1. Ask the volunteer to describe how she views or defines the problem. Help her conceptu-alize the essence of the problem and her goal.
2. Discuss with the volunteer what, if any, part of the problem she can do something about (i.e., control). Help her understand that different strategies should be generated for the parts she can control versus the parts she cannot control.
3. Once the situation has been defined, ask her (with the group's help) to generate alternative ways of responding to the situation. One alternative would be the client's typical response to the situation, which generally has more cons than pros or the issue would not still be a problem.
4. Determine with the volunteer (with the group's help) the full range of consequences that would result from each proposed alternative (i.e., positive and negative, both long- and short-term).
5. Help the volunteer group member select the most viable alternative (highest probability of gaining desired result) in collaboration with you and the group; elicit and integrate group members' perspectives here.
6. Have the volunteer make a commitment to implementing the chosen solution.

HANDOUT 11.1
Problem-Solving Method

Everyone has faced a problem or a decision that seemed impossible to deal with. Some people tend to get lost or stuck in emotions (anxiety, despair) around the problem—that's called "emotion-focused coping"—and do not find a solution. Other people experience and identify their emotions, but are then able to pivot to what's called "problem-focused coping," which is more effective than emotion-focused coping. One helpful type of problem-focused coping is a problem-solving method described here.

You may have used drinking to avoid dealing with problems; now you'll have an effective method to help resolve problems.

The problem-solving method has seven steps:

1. **Define the problem and your goal.** Think about the problem situation. Who is involved? When does it happen? Exactly what takes place? How does the problem affect you? What is the goal that you would like to achieve? **Be clear and specific**, not vague. **Define your goal as something that can be objectively evaluated.**

2. **Ask yourself, "Is there anything I can do about this?"** Is the problem (or any part of it) something you have any control over? If the problem is at least partially under your control, pick brainstorming options that involve a plan, approach, taking action, or fixing. If not under your control, choose brainstorming options that are focused on "how can I weather this or let it go for now" such as: acceptance/letting go, enlisting support, de-catastrophizing, using relaxation strategies, or talking about it with friend.

3. **Brainstorm for alternatives.** This can be a creative, fun step. *The goal of this step is to build a long list of possible solutions.* The first rule of brainstorming is that no idea is too silly or dumb. Try to think about any and every possible solution to the problem. Do not think about how good or bad each idea is—that will come later. *Don't skimp on the number of ideas you come up with.*

4. Now, **consider the consequences** of each. For each of your alternatives, list the pros and cons of each idea. Think about the short-term and long-term impact of each solution.

5. **Decide.** Which of the alternatives are the most likely to achieve the goal you set in Step 1? Look for the solution (or solutions) that has the best balance of pros and cons.

6. **Do it!** The best plan in the world is useless if you do not put it into action. Try it out.

7. **Evaluate.** Check out how the plan is working. Which parts work best? Which parts can you improve? Fix what can be fixed.

1. **Problem definition and goal**
   a. **Background:** Susan's live-in boyfriend is less responsible with money than she is, so she handles the accounting and also often pays all the household bills. She is developing resentment toward her boyfriend.
   b. **Goal:** Susan wants to find a different way to handle the accounting and make sure she and her boyfriend share expenses.

2. **What can and can't Susan control here?** Susan can control: her behavior, her suggestions, and the way she communicates and negotiates these suggestions to her boyfriend. She cannot control her boyfriend's emotional or verbal reactions.

3. **Brainstorming for alternatives**
   a. Keep doing the same thing—handle accounting, ask him for money when she needs it to pay bills, and hope he changes.
   b. Open a joint checking account into which their paychecks are direct-deposited, to use for the bills.
   c. Ask boyfriend to take over the bill-paying, and then he can ask her for her share.
   d. Hire an accountant or bookkeeper to handle and track all household finances.

4. Evaluate the pros and cons of each possible alternative:

	Pros	Cons
a. Keep doing same	+ Familiar + Boyfriend not mad	− Resentment grows − Possible break-up of relationship − Unfair to Susan
b. Open joint checking account	+ Fair to both + Susan doesn't have to ask boyfriend for money + Reduced resentment	− Need to deal with paperwork for direct deposit change
c. Ask boyfriend to take over bill-paying	+ Susan reduces resentment + Susan doesn't have to ask for money	− Boyfriend probably not capable − Damage to credit history − Bills not paid − Resentment increased
d. Hire accountant or bookkeeper	+ Less burden for Susan + Less resentment of boyfriend	− Expensive − Someone else knows all personal business

5. **Decide.** Opening a joint checking account seems like the best of these alternatives. Susan will need to talk with her boyfriend about this idea.

WORKSHEET 11.1
Problem-Solving

1. Define the problem and goal

   _____

   _____

   _____

2. Ask, "Is there anything I can do about this?" _____

3. Brainstorm for solutions and write them in the "Solutions" column below.

4. Evaluate the pros and cons of each solution and write them in the Pros and Cons columns below.

Solution	Pros	Cons
a.		
b.		
c.		
d.		
e.		

5. Pick solution(s): _____

6. Implement the solution for a period of time.

7. Re-evaluate the solution. Did it work? If not, do problem-solving again.

Catch Up on Prior Session Material, Review and Consolidate What Has Been Covered So Far (10 minutes)

Use this time to open discussion to catch up on unfinished material from previous sessions, to clarify anything covered in previous sessions, and/or to review/discuss what has been especially helpful so far and in what way.

Farewell to Members Leaving the Group (10 minutes)

Have members who are leaving identify the skills they think have been most important to the changes that they have made during therapy, i.e., those skills they will continue to try to implement in order to maintain their progress. Remind group members that relapses most often occur in the types of situations they are now prepared to handle.

For women finishing the group, ask them how they feel about finishing the treatment program. Explore termination issues—fear, relief, loss. Discuss referrals for additional treatment if necessary. Discuss the possibility that group members may wish to stay in contact and provide support to one another.

Each group member who is finishing treatment should also be asked to go around the room and say something positive or constructive to each of her fellow group members. These statements could focus on positive changes or steps the leaving group member has seen each of the other women make during treatment, or ways in which the leaving group member feels she herself has learned or benefited from other women in the group. Other group members also should be encouraged to give some positive feedback to the woman who is finishing treatment. Women who are finishing treatment and the therapist may also want to say something to one another.

Anticipating High-Risk Situations This Week (10 minutes)

Rationale:

At the end of each session, we will spend a bit of time discussing any problem situations that each member thinks might come up around drinking or drug use this week. As you each progress through therapy, you will get better and better at anticipating and handling these. A "high-risk situation" is a situation in which you would find it very difficult not to drink. Today, I'd like us each to spend a few minutes together thinking about the upcoming week. [For each group member:] *Are there any situations that you might encounter this week that would tempt you to drink or use drugs?*

EXERCISE 11.2
High-Risk Situations and Executing High-Risk Situation Plans

Use Worksheet 11.2: High-Risk Situations, located in the Client Workbook Worksheet 11.2:

Now let's each use Worksheet 11.2: High-Risk Situations to write in a high-risk situation for this upcoming week and brainstorm together about strategies/solutions you can use to cope with that high-risk situation in order to avoid drinking or using drugs in response to it. Are there any situations that you might encounter this week that would tempt you to drink or use drugs?

Elicit examples of upcoming high-risk situations from members and brainstorm together to generate plans for how to handle the situation for two or three group members. Write ideas about how to handle this situation on the High-Risk Situations worksheet. Refer to Session 1 in this guide for a copy of the worksheet or to the Client Workbook for a client version of the worksheet.

Assign Homework (5 minutes)

Here is a list of homework assignments for each group member to complete between today's session and the next. Remind the women how important it is to complete the homework.

1. Complete one self-monitoring card each day.
2. On the back of your self-monitoring cards, write down high-risk situations you encountered and how you handled them.
3. Read all the Session 11 material in your workbook and complete worksheets you didn't finish during the session.
4. Complete one problem-solving exercise at home.
5. Complete Worksheet 11.2: High-Risk Situations, located in the Client Workbook, and execute high-risk situation plans.

CHAPTER 17

Session 12: Relapse Prevention II, Maintenance Planning

(Corresponds to Chapter 12 in the Client Workbook)
(1.5 hours)

Notes to the Therapist Before the Session

1. For rolling-admission groups (see Chapter 3), each new member should have an individual assessment (see Chapter 5) with the group facilitator prior to joining the group. At the end of the assessment session, for women joining the group at any session (i.e., Session 2–12) after Session 1, the therapist should spend an additional 30 minutes with each new group member to provide the Client Workbook and to review basic information covered in Session 1 that the client will need to know to proceed with all subsequent sessions. This includes coverage of use of the Client Workbook and group rules, as well as a brief review of core treatment elements, including self-monitoring, psychoeducation, high-risk situations, triggers, and behavior chains (see Session 2). That way, no matter what session the new member is entering, she will be able to do daily self-monitoring and understand the basics of high-risk situations, triggers, and behavior chains.

2. Each rolling-admission group session with a new member starts with a 5-minute round robin introduction of each group member, and 10 minutes of assessment feedback to the new member(s) (see Session 1 for detailed instructions and feedback sheets). Members in the group at different stages of recovery can provide support to the new client and share their own feedback from their first session. If a new member is lacking relevant information from previous sessions, she can review sessions in the Client Workbook or you can briefly describe the

section, and/or abstinent members can be encouraged to spend time with the new member after session to explain relevant prior material.

3. For each new member entering the group in Sessions 2 to 12, follow instructions at the beginning of each session regarding Introductions and Providing Assessment Feedback in Client's First Session.

4. If this is a client's first session, you must summarize data from the pretreatment assessment to fill in a Feedback Sheet (see Handout 1.10 in Client Workbook) for each client in the group in preparation for her first session.

5. Before the session begins, write the session agenda on a flipchart, whiteboard, or blackboard.

6. If you are doing the Optional Graphing Intervention, see instructions in Chapter 3 of this Therapist Guide.

7. All worksheets and handouts used in this treatment program appear in this Therapist Guide and in the corresponding Client Workbook; worksheets (and selected handouts) can also be accessed by searching for this book's title on the Oxford Academic platform, at academic. oup.com.

Session 12 Outline

All times are approximate and should be adjusted based on clinical need and whether group time needs to be devoted to new or departing members.

1. Pre-session sign-in and substance use check (15 minutes before session begins)
2. Introductions and agenda setting (5 minutes)
3. Check-in, review of self-monitoring and homework (15 minutes)
4. Relapse prevention II: Identifying and managing warning signs of relapse, handling slips or relapses (40 minutes)
5. Relapse contract (15 minutes)
6. Farewell to members leaving the group (10 minutes)
7. Anticipating high-risk situations this week (5 minutes)
8. Assign homework (5 minutes)

1. Flipchart, whiteboard, or blackboard, felt-tip markers or chalk, eraser
2. Breathalyzer and tubes or saliva strips (optional)
3. Saliva drug tests for each group member (optional)
4. Seven self-monitoring cards for each group member (Note to therapist: Keep a stack of these to give group members at each session.)
5. OPTIONAL: Individualized graph for each woman
6. Handouts
    12.1: Slips and Relapses
    12.2: Warning Signs of Slips or Relapse
    12.3: Handling Slips and Relapses
    12.4: Plan for Handling Slips and Relapses—Example
    12.5: Relapse Contract—Sample
7. Worksheets
    12.1: Identifying and Managing Slip and Relapse Warning Signs
    12.2: Plan for Handling Slips and Relapses
    12.3: Relapse Contract
    12.4: High-Risk Situations [See Client Workbook Worksheet 12.4]

If any member of the group appears to be high or intoxicated, you may want to assess her blood alcohol level (BAL) with a breathalyzer or saliva strip or use a saliva drug screen. Regardless of formal testing, though, if a group member is visibly high or intoxicated, review the treatment agreement with her and let her know that she will not be allowed to attend this session. Clients who miss a session will not receive a make-up session, but encourage them to read the handouts they missed for that session and complete the homework for the following week. You should assist the client in arranging alternate transportation home, review her abstinence plan, and remind her of her abstinence goal.

Introductions and Agenda Setting (5 minutes)

You will introduce new members joining the group this session, and provide an overview (i.e., set agenda) of what will be covered in the session. The purpose of Session 12 is to focus on maintenance of change in drinking or drug use and to provide relapse prevention skills. Ask the group if there is anything pressing they would like to discuss today in addition to the planned material. Explain the absence of missing members without revealing protected health information.

Check-In, Review of Self-Monitoring and Homework (15 minutes)

Check-in follows a "round robin" format, in which drinking status and homework are emphasized. To introduce the round robin check-in:

We're going to go around the room using what we call a "round robin check-in" to get a brief version of how your week has been, focusing on your alcohol use, drug use, cravings, and triggers; how you coped with triggers and cravings; in hindsight what you might have done differently (with therapist and group input/ideas as well); homework you completed and what was helpful about it. We also will answer or clarify any questions or concerns about the homework material. Each group member will have a few minutes [depending on how many women there are in the group] *to discuss with the group how your coping with alcohol/drug use triggers has been this week.*

> **Therapist Note**
> *Try to pay particular attention to women's specific themes (e.g., right to self-care, empowerment) to link experiences to the specific theme: "One theme I've heard that's common among several of you is . . ."*

Go around the room and ask each group member how her week was (focusing on alcohol and/or drug use); listen while looking over her self-monitoring cards; and link what she is saying to her daily cards for alcohol/drug cravings, triggers, and use. Use information from this for specific topics in the rest of the session. Check in with each group member and discuss the progress of her abstinence plan. Update the plan if necessary. Also remember to ask each client at the end of her round robin time about what homework she was able to complete.

You should reinforce self-recording behavior, check for questions or problems, and help group members develop solutions for difficulties related to self-recording procedures. Ask members if they have any questions. Possible questions to anticipate include:

▪ **Question:** I thought about drinking the whole morning. Is that one urge or more than one?

THERAPIST: *You had the urge continually?*

CLIENT: Not every minute.

THERAPIST: *Well, each time you have a thought or an image about having a specific type of drink or a drink in a particular situation, that counts as a separate urge. Can you share some specific situations you thought about?*

▪ **Question:** Why are my urges so much higher than everyone else's? Why am I the only one still drinking?

THERAPIST: *It's natural that you would want to compare your drinking/ drug use and urges to those of the other group members. Although this can be an important motivator, it also is important to remember that everyone has her own unique path to abstinence. You're working on it, so be patient with yourself, and think of the changes you've already made! What does the group think about what _____ said?*

Therapist Note
After reviewing the daily monitoring cards, for outpatient settings you may wish to include the optional Graphing Intervention here.

Optional Graphing Intervention for Outpatient Treatment Settings

See the detailed instructions in Chapter 3 of this guide for how to use the graphs located in Session 2 of the Therapist Guide and in the Client Workbook (Handout 2.1. Graph: Alcohol/Drug Use and Urges Sample and Worksheet 2.1. Graph: Alcohol/Drug Use and Urges). This intervention will allow each woman to track her progress by entering weekly data summarized from her daily monitoring cards: 1. Number of drinks; 2. Number of drugs used; 3. Number of urges/cravings; and 4. Average strength of urges/cravings.

Other Homework Review

Review all other homework clients did during the prior week. Reinforce clients for completing homework and discuss barriers experienced in completing the homework. Ask questions such as, *"What did you learn from the homework?"* or *"How can you use the homework to help you in the future?"*

Remember that as part of homework review, each week you need to review group members' recording of high-risk situations and how these were handled: *"Who wants to share how you handled one of your high-risk situations this week without drinking/using drugs?"* Elicit high-risk examples from two or three group members and get feedback from other members. Remember to have group members direct their comments to the other group members, and not just to you. Point out common types of high-risk situations among the group members and encourage women facing similar situations to share how they coped or ideas for coping. Selectively model and repeat empowering and motivational positive affirmations that group members give to one another: for example, *"We know this is hard, you're doing great." "Next time you'll be able to use a different strategy, hang in there."*

Also, ask about progress with doctor's appointments and blood tests. Due to time constraints, group members should discuss any concerns about their blood test or feedback with you after the group. Ask each client to bring in a copy of her lab results and give it to you. You can give feedback to the client during review of homework either that week or the week after.

> **Therapist Note**
> *You should manage participation so that there is enough time to go around the room in a round robin fashion and give each group member a chance to speak. Keep in mind that 10 to 30 minutes total is allotted for check-in depending on how many women are in the group. If homework*

> *is not done, you should ask what made it difficult for the client to complete the homework. The importance of completing homework should be discussed, and a firm commitment for the future should be stressed in a nonjudgmental way.*

Share the following with the group:

> *The time in the treatment group is only part of the process. The real change occurs when you practice changing your lives in the real world. The group will help you get ideas, stay motivated, keep you on track, and develop an understanding of the problem. But actually changing behavior takes place in your everyday life—at home, at work, with family, friends, and so on.*

> **Therapist Note**
> *The following are some tips for managing members' participation to maintain the temporal structure of the session: For habitually quiet members or those who appear upset or distressed, you should acknowledge them with empathic nonverbal behavior, but do not call on them to elicit participation right away, except during their turn in the round robin. Look for opportunities to invite limited participation of habitually quiet members to help them become comfortable sharing. Frequently ask the group for their feedback on particular group members' contributions, to set up the expectation that group members will be doing a lot of the work in the room. Everyone in the group learns by hearing the experiences and advice of others. Model and facilitate a tone of supportive, constructive, and compassionate feedback in the group. Don't be confrontational, but also don't condone or reassure a woman about her drinking/drug use or lack of work outside the group sessions. For instance, don't say, "It's okay. You had a really hard week; of course you drank a bit." Say instead, "You certainly had a hard week! In hindsight, what could you have done differently in response to trigger xxx?"*

Group members who are having substantial difficulty with their abstinence plan or who appear to be at risk for an emergency should be asked discreetly to remain after group for an individual check-in with you.

Relapse Prevention II: Identifying and Managing Warning Signs of Relapse, Handling Slips or Relapses (40 minutes)

Rationale:

The focus of our treatment has been on helping you achieve abstinence and developing the skills you need to maintain abstinence in the long run. It may seem pessimistic to discuss drinking or drug use when you're not using, but we like to think about relapse prevention the way we think about fire prevention—it is necessary to examine your home or workplace to try to eliminate fire hazards, and it's also necessary to have a fire extinguisher, fire drill, phone number of the fire department, and so on, in case something unexpected happens. It's a safety net.

*Also, because of the nature of alcohol and other substance use disorders, we do know that many people who **want to stay sober** still have difficulties at times, and they may experience a slip or relapse. We want to help you be prepared for situations you may face after this treatment program is over.*

We will be focusing on relapses in three ways—by helping you identify warning signs of slips and relapses, by developing strategies to avoid slips or relapses, and by developing strategies to cope with slips or relapses should they occur.

Psychoeducation on Slips and Relapses, Warning Signs of Slips and Relapses, Handling Slips and Relapses

Review Handout 12.1: Slips and Relapses with the group. Generate discussion.

Then review Handout 12.2: Warning Signs of Slips or Relapse. Generate discussion. Do Exercise 12.1., Identifying and Managing Warning signs, using Worksheet 12.1.

Then do Exercise 12.2., Handling Slips and Relapses, using Handout 12.3: Handling Slips and Relapses, and Handout 12.4: Plan for Handling Slips and Relapses—Example, and Worksheet 12.2.

Helpful Ways to Think About Slips and Relapses

A **slip** is a one-time event, an initial return to drinking or drug use (one or two drinks or one drug use occasion, or 1 or 2 days of drinking or using). It is a *mistake* that should not be repeated.

❖ A slip is an *opportunity* to learn about something risky. You can think of different ways to handle the same situation in the future. *Message:* You do NOT need to continue drinking/drug use and you can learn a lesson for the future, which will make you stronger/more resilient.

❖ The slip is a NOT a *disaster* and doesn't mean that you are hopeless. Some people, if they slip, think things like "I have blown it. I will never succeed. I will just give up." (**This type of thinking is NOT helpful. This is called "catastrophizing."**)

❖ **Other people may catastrophize about your slip, thinking or saying things like:** "She will never get better." "Here we go again." "All that money and time for nothing." "I knew it. I can never trust her." "Treatment was a failure." These thoughts and words are NOT helpful, but you should not expect your family to understand completely. Remind yourself that their reaction is normal and comes from anxiety about a possible return to drinking or drug use. Try not to get angry; say you understand why they might be feeling this way and ask how you can help to reassure them.

❖ Slips are like falling off a bicycle. You don't want to or intend to fall, but you might. A fall may hurt, but you should get back on the bicycle and keep riding. You may feel rotten about the slip, but you can learn from it. However, even one slip can start a "slippery slope" leading to additional use of alcohol or drugs—in the same week, or the following weeks, and gradually escalating over subsequent weeks. So, it is important to try to avoid slips, to acknowledge what you could have done differently to not drink/use in the "slip" situation, and to plan for future similar situations.

A **relapse** is a return to regular, heavy, problem drinking or drug use in the same pattern you had before you sought treatment. **The typical road to recovery is a bumpy one.** Many women feel shame about slipping or relapsing. They believe that most other people just stop drinking/using drugs and it's a straight road to eternal abstinence. That is not a realistic way to think about an alcohol use disorder or other substance use disorder. It is typically a bumpy road, and though slips along the way are not desired or the goal, they can happen, and the best thing to do is to not think of one as a disaster or a catastrophe. A time-limited slip does NOT need to continue into a full-blown relapse. A slip is a mistake that can be fixed right away and is an opportunity for growth. Even a relapse is not a catastrophe—you can work with your therapist or support network to stop it, learn from it, and get back on track. The ultimate goal is long-term abstinence.

❖ **A good safeguard: Learn to identify warning signs of a slip or a relapse.** Prepare a plan in advance to deal with the warning signs so that you can avoid a slip or relapse. Prepare a plan in advance to cope with a slip, should it happen, so you can return to abstinence right away. Even prepare a plan in advance to cope with a relapse, should it happen.

HANDOUT 12.2
Warning Signs of Slips or Relapse

❖ We know that many women who *want to stay sober* may have difficulties from time to time. An important skill is to be aware of warning signs and take steps to address the signs so that you don't end up drinking or using drugs again.

❖ We want you to think about *warning signs* of a slip or relapse. It's like fire prevention. For fire prevention, we look at possible dangers in our homes, schools, and workplaces. We know where to find the fire extinguishers and how to contact the fire department. We remain aware of possible trouble: something flammable near a heat source or strange smoke. Similarly, we should remain aware of signs of trouble about possible drinking or using and have a plan in place.

❖ **Warning signs might be changes in the way you think, or changes in your behaviors or habits.** Warning signs also include an increase in the frequency or intensity of cravings to drink or use drugs. You have learned many new behaviors in this program. Through dedication, these behaviors can become everyday habits. Changes in these new habits may signal trouble. Keep an eye out for old habits, ones that led to trouble in the past. Try to be in touch with changes in mood, people you associate with, places you go, ways you handle problems, and your routines. Be alert for changes in the way you think about alcohol, drugs, yourself, or things around you. **Any of these could signal the possibility of a slip. Women tend to slip in response to a variety of triggers: interaction with drinkers or drug users in their social network, the availability of alcohol or drugs, negative emotions, shame, and social anxiety. Premenstrual emotionality may be a trigger for some women.**

❖ **Think back to your last slips.** What were the signals of trouble? Remember the few days before the slip. What things had changed? Look for changes in your actions or thoughts that may have warned you of trouble. **These old signals are ones you should watch for.** Here's an example of how to think about and plan for warning signs:

Warning Signs for a Slip or Relapse	How to Handle Warning Signs
1. Isolating: keeping to myself and not going out with friends	1. For every night that I find myself isolating, make plans to see friends.
2. Skipping more than 1 day at the gym	2. Keep track of gym days on my calendar, take note at the end of each week.
3. Not getting 8 hours of sleep each night	3. Ask Maria to watch TV in the den at night—it keeps me awake in the bedroom.
4. Lying to Maria about how I'm feeling, going back to "Oh, I'm fine!"	4. Ask Maria to call me out—keep working on our communication, I'm worth it.
5. Going to Danielle's house	5. Think about the long-term consequences. Re-read my "reasons for quitting" list!

EXERCISE 12.1
Identifying and Managing Warning Signs

In this exercise, you will help clients identify their own warning signs for relapse. For this exercise, you will be using Handout 12.2: Warning Signs of Slips or Relapse and Worksheet 12.1: Identifying and Managing Slip and Relapse Warning Signs.

Now, we will work together to develop our own list of slip and relapse warning signs and how to handle them.

Ask for a volunteer to go through this exercise with you while you write her answers on the whiteboard/flipchart. The rest of the group should contribute ideas and observations while also starting to fill out their own Worksheet 12.1.

To the volunteer:

Think back to the last relapse that you experienced—what kinds of thoughts, feelings, or behaviors occurred before the slip or relapse that could have been warning signs that a relapse might be coming? We'll be using Worksheet 12.1. Everyone else can follow along, writing down your own warning signs.

Ask the volunteer to think about the days and weeks before the relapse and identify changes in her usual thoughts, habits, and moods; the people with whom she was spending time; the places she visited; the ways that she handled problems or stressors, etc. Using the whiteboard/flipchart, write a list of the warning signs that the volunteer describes. Also, elicit additional suggestions from the group.

Does anyone else want to share the kinds of thoughts, feelings, or behaviors that occurred right before your own slips/relapses so that we can start to come up with a list of your warning signs?

You can also point out that group members have learned new ways of coping during therapy, so *not* using those new coping strategies might also be a warning sign. For example, one client might have initiated a regular exercise program after work at a time when she previously drank or used. Stopping the exercise program, or beginning to skip workouts, might be a subtle warning sign for impending relapse because she would be beginning to fall back into her old patterns. You should also refer to the notion of "seemingly irrelevant decisions" introduced in Session 10—these are changes in patterns that *seem* to have nothing to do with drinking or drug use, but that in fact set the client up to drink or use.

WORKSHEET 12.1
Identifying and Managing Slip and Relapse Warning Signs

Warning Signs for a Slip or Relapse

How to Handle Warning Signs

1. _____

1. _____

_____

_____

2. _____

2. _____

_____

_____

3. _____

3. _____

_____

_____

4. _____

4. _____

_____

_____

5. _____

5. _____

_____

_____

EXERCISE 12.2
Handling Slips and Relapses

For this exercise, you will help clients develop plans for handling potential slips or relapses. You will use Handouts 12.3: Handling Slips and Relapses and 12.4: Plan for Handling Slips and Relapses—Example and Worksheet 12.2: Plan for Handling Slips and Relapses.

Now, we will talk about what to do if you actually do slip (drink or use drugs) or relapse back to your prior heavy pattern of use. Let's review together Handout 12.3: Handling Slips and Relapses. Then together we will go through Handout 12.4: Plan for Handling Slips and Relapses—Example; this is a sample worksheet to provide some ideas. After that, we will work through Worksheet 12.2: Plan for Handling Slips and Relapses with a volunteer, while everyone also starts to fill in their own Worksheet 12.2.

HANDOUT 12.3
Handling Slips and Relapses

It is important that you have tools to handle slips and relapses.

Looking for and thinking about warning signs help to prevent a slip. However, even people who work hard to remain abstinent may find themselves in an overwhelming situation. While you should work hard and expect to not use alcohol or drugs again, you still should be prepared to handle a slip in a problem-focused way, without falling into despair or shame, which would just set you up to drink or use drugs more.

If you do have a drink or use drugs, remember the following. A slip often precedes a relapse, and without a slip there would have been no progression to relapse. Thus, most of these suggestions focus on handling a slip.

1. **Don't panic.** One drink/drug occasion does not have to lead to an extended binge, or to a return to uncontrolled use.
2. **Stop, look, and listen.** *Stop* the ongoing flow of events and *look and listen* to what is happening (do a behavior chain). The slip should be seen as a warning signal that you are in trouble. The slip is like a flat tire—it's time to pull off the road to deal with the situation.
3. **Be aware of the "abstinence violation effect."** Once you have a drink/use drugs, you may have thoughts such as "I blew it," "All my efforts were a waste," "As long as I've blown it, I might as well keep using," "My willpower has failed. I have no control," or "I'm an addict and I can't control it." These thoughts might be accompanied by feelings of anger or guilt. It is crucial to dispute these thoughts immediately.
4. **Renew your commitment.** After a slip, it is easy to feel discouraged and to want to give up. Think back over the reasons why you decided to change your drinking/drug use in the first place. Think about all the positive long-term benefits of abstinence and the long-term problems associated with continued use.
5. **Decide on a course of action.** At a minimum, this should include the following:
   - Get out of the drinking/drug use situation.
   - Wait at least 2 hours before having a second drink or another use of drug.
   - During those 2 hours, engage in some activity that would help you avoid continued drinking/drug use. Review materials from treatment, talk over the slip with someone who could be helpful, or call your therapist.
   - Make an appointment with a therapist as soon as possible to get back on track.
   - Tell someone! Once it's "public" it will be easier to not progress and to seek help. Ask for help.
6. **Review the situation leading up to the slip.** Take responsibility and learn from your mistakes, but don't beat yourself up for what happened. Ask yourself the following:
   - What events led up to the slip?
   - What were the main triggers?
   - Were there any early warning signs?
   - Did you try to deal with these constructively?
   - If not, why not? Was your motivation weakened by fatigue, social pressure, depression?

Once you have analyzed the slip, think about what changes you need to make to avoid future slips.

HANDOUT 12.4
Plan for Handling Slips and Relapses—Example

Immediate plans to prevent the slip from becoming a relapse:

Remember that my judgment is impaired now because I had a drink. I just need to leave the situation and get away from alcohol availability, or dump out the rest of the wine.

Call or text my partner/family.
Call my therapist or my AA sponsor.

Use paced breathing, pour myself a nonalcoholic beverage, and take a walk.
Go to sleep or take a nap.
Call my therapist to arrange a session ASAP.

How I will get support to handle the relapse:

Talk to Sam (partner) about any relapses/slips rather than trying to hide it from him.

Discuss slips, relapses, and urges with my therapist or sponsor or group member.

Maintain my relationship with AA sponsor for help with relapse—tell her as soon as possible.

Try naltrexone to stop myself from having cravings in the next few days/week. Call my psychiatrist or get a referral to an addiction physician to prescribe.

Going forward . . .

Get back on track with my new routine.
Address increased depression with my therapist.

Resume going to meetings regularly, or start/resume therapy.

Write down positive thoughts about how the slip doesn't have to be a relapse. Focus on what to do differently next time.
Sign up for a new exercise class.

WORKSHEET 12.2
Plan for Handling Slips and Relapses

Immediate plans to prevent the slip from becoming a relapse:

_____

_____

_____

_____

How I will get support to handle a relapse:

_____

_____

_____

_____

Going forward . . .

_____

_____

_____

_____

EXERCISE 12.3
Write a Relapse Contract

For this exercise, you will help group members develop a personal contract for steps they will commit to take if they experience a slip or relapse. You will be using Handout 12.5: Relapse Contract—Sample and Worksheet 12.3: Relapse Contract.

Explain the purpose of the relapse contract described in Handout 12.5. Work out a personalized relapse contract with a volunteer client (if possible choose a group member who is at the end of or finishing the treatment soon), while other members watch and contribute their ideas to the plan. You do *not* need to exactly follow the sample as if it is a template—this is just an example for the level of detail that is typically most helpful. Include ways to address the possible relapse warning signs and ways of handling those that the volunteer has identified. Conduct a round robin review with each client who is finishing treatment with this session, to discuss her relapse contract. Have each group member sign her contract. For clients not ending with this session, have them complete a draft relapse contract that they will revisit at their own last treatment session.

Relapse Contract—Sample (for client who does not use drugs)

1. If I drink any alcohol in the next 6 months, I will sit down the following day and strategize what to do to prevent this slip from becoming a full-blown relapse using Worksheet 12.2: Plan for Handling Slips and Relapses. I will also complete a behavior chain worksheet to figure out what happened. I will call or text Susan, my best friend, to tell her and ask for support or help. I also will contact my therapist right away to set up a booster session appointment. If my provider recommends a higher level of care, I will consider that.

2. If, within 1 month of drinking, I drink again (even 1 standard drink), I will begin/resume regular weekly treatment with a therapist. I will also call a medical provider to discuss the use of an anti-craving or other type of medication. I will also take every other step I listed above in #1.

3. If I binge-drink (more than 3 standard drinks on any one occasion) even once, I will contact a therapist to resume or begin weekly sessions, and I will tell Susan and my brother. I will also take every other step I listed above in #1.

4. After 6 months, I will re-evaluate this contract and write a new one.

_____   _____

Client   Date

_____   _____

Witness (Therapist)   Date

WORKSHEET 12.3
Relapse Contract

1. If I drink any alcohol or use any _____ (name of drug) in the next ____ months, I will

_____

_____

_____

2. If within _____ week/month of drinking or using a drug, I drink again (even 1 standard drink) or use _____ (drug) even once, I will

_____

_____

_____

3. If I binge-drink (more than ___ standard drinks on any one occasion) even once, _____

_____

_____

_____

4. After ___ months, I will re-evaluate this contract and write a new one.

_____   _____

Client   Date

_____   _____

Witness (Therapist)   Date

Farewell to Members Leaving the Group (10 minutes)

Have members who are leaving identify the skills they think have been most important to the changes that they have made during therapy, i.e., those skills they will continue to try to implement in order to maintain their progress. Remind group members that relapses most often occur in the types of situations they are now prepared to handle.

For women finishing the group, ask them how they feel about finishing the treatment program. Explore termination issues—fear, relief, loss. Discuss referrals for additional treatment if necessary. Discuss the possibility that group members may wish to stay in contact and provide support to one another.

Each group member who is finishing treatment should also be asked to go around the room and say something positive or constructive to each of her fellow group members. These statements could focus on positive changes or steps the leaving group member has seen each of the other women make during treatment, or ways in which the leaving group member feels she herself has learned or benefited from other women in the group. Other group members also should be encouraged to give some positive feedback to the woman who is finishing treatment. Women who are finishing treatment and the therapist may also want to say something to one another.

Anticipating High-Risk Situations This Week (5 minutes)

Rationale:

At the end of each session, we will spend a bit of time discussing any problem situations that each member thinks might come up around drinking or drug use this week. As you each progress through therapy, you will get better and better at anticipating and handling these. A "high-risk situation" is a situation in which you would find it very difficult not to drink. Today, I'd like us each to spend a few minutes together thinking about the upcoming week. [For each group member:] Are there any situations that you might encounter this week that would tempt you to drink or use drugs?

EXERCISE 12.4
High-Risk Situations and Executing High-Risk Situation Plans

Use Worksheet 12.4: High-Risk Situations, located in the Client Workbook:

Now let's each use Worksheet 12.4: High-Risk Situations to write in a high-risk situation for this upcoming week and brainstorm together about strategies/solutions you can use to cope with that high-risk situation in order to avoid drinking or using drugs in response to it. Are there any situations that you might encounter this week that would tempt you to drink or use drugs?

Elicit examples of upcoming high-risk situations from members and brainstorm together to generate plans for how to handle the situation for two or three group members. Write ideas about how to handle this situation on the High-Risk Situations worksheet. Refer to Session 1 in this guide for a copy of the worksheet or to the Client Workbook Worksheet 12.4: High-Risk Situations. for a client version of the worksheet.

Assign Homework (5 minutes)

Here is a list of homework assignments for each group member to complete between today's session and the next. Remind the women how important it is to complete the homework.

1. Complete one self-monitoring card each day.
2. On the back of your self-monitoring cards, write down high-risk situations you encountered and how you handled them.
3. Read all the Session 12 material in your workbook and complete worksheets you didn't finish during the session.
4. Complete Worksheet 12.4: High-Risk Situations, located in the Client Workbook, and execute high-risk situation plans.

Self-Report Measures

A. Combined Drinker Inventory of Consequences (DrINC) and Inventory of Drug Use Consequences (InDUC)

A combined version of the DrINC and InDUC can be found at:

Questionnaire: InDUC-2L.pdf (unm.edu)

Scoring sheet: InDUC Scoring Sheet.pdf (unm.edu)

Psychometric articles: https://casaa.unm.edu/inst/inducpa.html

B. Personal Drinking or Drug Use Goal

Please read the goals listed below and choose the one that best represents your thoughts about drinking and drug use at this time by circling the number that corresponds to your goal.

1. I have decided not to change my pattern of drinking or drug use.
2. Fill in a, b, or both if this is the choice you are thinking about:
   a. I have decided to cut down on my drinking and drink in a more controlled manner—to be in control of how often I drink and how much I drink. I would like to limit myself to no more than _____ drinks per _____ (days, weeks, or months).
   b. I have decided to cut down on my drug use and use in a more controlled manner. I would like to limit myself to no more than _____ amount of _____ (name the drugs) per _____ (days, weeks, or months).
3. I have decided to stop drinking and using drugs completely for a period of time, after which I will make a new decision about whether I will drink/use again. For me, the period of time I want to stop drinking/using drugs is _____ (days, weeks, months, years).
4. I have decided to stop drinking or using drugs regularly, but would like to have an occasional drink or use a drug when I really have the urge.
5. I have decided to quit drinking or using drugs once and for all, even though I realize I may slip up and drink or use drugs once in a while.
6. I have decided to quit drinking and using drugs once and for all, to be totally abstinent, and never drink alcohol or use drugs ever again for the rest of my life.
7. None of this applies exactly to me. My own goal is: _____
   (Adapted from Hall et al., 1991)

C. Psychiatric Symptom Screening Measures

Alternative Psychiatric Screening Measures:

1. **Beck Depression Inventory:** BDI-II Beck Depression Inventory-II (pearsonassessments. com). From the website: "The Beck Depression Inventory®-II is a brief, self-report inventory designed to measure the severity of depression symptomatology."

2. **Burns Anxiety Inventory:** Burns_Anxiety_Inventory (vpweb.com). Brief self-report inventory of recent anxiety symptoms.

3. **American Psychiatric Association DSM-5 screener:** DSM5 Self-Rated Level 1 Cross-Cutting Symptom Measure.pdf (cimpress.io). Per the American Psychiatric Association: "This material can be reproduced without permission by researchers and by clinicians for use with their patients."

4. **OQ-45.2:** OQ®-45.2-OQ Measures (Outcome Questionnaire OQ-45: Fill and Sign Printable Template Online [uslegalforms.com]). From the website: "Designed for on-going measurement of client progress throughout therapy and following termination, the OQ®-45.2 is the adult outcome measure of choice by the Canadian government, and one of America's largest health care systems, as well as an entire branch of the U.S. Armed Services."

5. **PCL-5 (PTSD symptom checklist)** (Weathers et al., 2013). Brief measure of PTSD symptoms, not used to establish a diagnosis. Can be obtained at PTSD Checklist for DSM-5 (PCL-5)—PTSD: National Center for PTSD (va.gov) for the measure, interpretation of scores, and limitations on use.

D. Current Medications

Are you currently taking medication to treat a psychological/psychiatric or a medical problem? (Yes / No)

If yes, please list the names, dosage, and dates of your current medications:

Rx Name: _____Dosage:___mg Start Date:___/____/_____

Rx Name: _____Dosage:___mg Start Date:___/____/_____

Rx Name: _____Dosage:___mg Start Date:___/____/_____

Rx Name: _____Dosage:___mg Start Date:___/____/_____

Rx Name: _____Dosage:___mg Start Date:___/____/_____

Rx Name: _____Dosage:___mg Start Date:___/____/_____

E. Hospitalizations

Have you ever been hospitalized for a psychiatric or addiction problem? (Yes / No). If yes, please

complete the information below:

Hospital	Year	# of Days	Reason(s)
_____	_____	_____	_____
_____	_____	_____	_____
_____	_____	_____	_____
_____	_____	_____	_____
_____	_____	_____	_____
_____	_____	_____	_____
_____	_____	_____	_____

F. Family Psychiatric and Addiction History

(For biological relatives. If adopted, please put "A" next to your parents' names and list anything you know about your biological relatives and also about your adoptive family.)

Relationship to You (*Please list name*)	Living / Deceased (*If deceased, year of death*)	Age	Mental Health Issues / Psychiatric Diagnoses / Alcohol or Substance Use Disorder (*Please describe*)
Mother			
Father			
Sibling			
Sibling			
Sibling			
Stepmother			
Stepfather			
Half-/step-sibling			
Half-/step-sibling			

Clinical Intake Interview

Note: If possible, the clinical intake interview should be conducted after the client has filled out self-report forms and the therapist has reviewed the forms.

Therapist introduction:

This is a semi-structured clinical interview to learn about your history of and recent drug and alcohol use and related problems, as well as additional information that will be helpful for treatment planning. For some of the questions, I'll be looking for specific yes/no answers and I'll ask for additional information if need be. Some questions will be more open-ended. I would like to get an initial sense of your situation without going into too much detail at this time, and we'll have plenty of time to go into more detail over the next few weeks. This interview should be about 90 minutes and includes some questionnaires for you to complete afterwards (if you haven't already), for our use in sessions going forward.

A. Clinical Questions About Nature of the Problem (10–15 minutes)

1. *What have been the main difficulties that led to your seeking treatment at this time?* If not clear, query for primary substance of choice/abuse—i.e., *Which drug (and/or alcohol) would you say is causing the most problems currently? What problems has the drinking/drug use caused?*

_____

_____

_____

_____

_____

_____

2. *Are there any additional concerns, problems, or behaviors that you have been struggling with, or issues/relationships you think have been problematic (e.g., mood swings, trauma history, eating disorder, depression, anxiety, unhealthy relationships)?*

_____

_____

_____

_____

_____

_____

3. *How are you feeling right now?*

_____

_____

_____

_____

B. Current Problem Substances

Enter one substance per line—alcohol and/or drugs.

1. _____

2. _____

3. _____

4. _____

5. _____

C. Overview Questions About Alcohol and Drug Use

1. *When did you last have a drink of alcohol or use a drug?* (month, day, time of day)

_____

2. *What and how much did you drink or use at that time?*

_____

3. *When and what did you drink or use the time before that (and the time before that, etc.)?*

_____

4. *How many years has drinking or drug use been a problem for you?*

_____

D. Current/Recent Alcohol/Drug Use

1. *Over the past month or so, how many days per week have you had any alcohol to drink? What about other drugs?*

_____

2. *What do you like to drink?*

_____

3. *Approximately how much do you usually drink?*

_____

4. *What is the typical amount you use of* _____ *(drug of choice)?*

_____

5. *How long have you been drinking/using drugs in this pattern?* (Get typical pattern of quantity/frequency in standard drinks—briefly.)

_____

6. If the client has not had a drink or used any drugs in the past month or has been drinking or using drugs at a lower level than previously in an effort to cut down, ask about the pattern of the last month and then ask again for the most recent pattern of problematic drinking or drug use. You may use the following questions:

a. *How many months/years did you drink/use drugs in this general pattern?*

_____

b. *What was your drinking/drug use pattern like before that and how long did it last?*

_____

c. *When was the last time you drank/used drugs?*

_____

E. Quantity/Frequency of Use of Each Substance: Lifetime Drug Use Chart

I'd like to get a more specific understanding of your drug and alcohol use over your lifetime using this chart we can fill out together.

- Instructions for administration of Table A.1:
  - First ask the Question 1 for each drug in the column and get a yes/no answer for each category.
  - For each drug used, circle or write in the specific drug used.
  - For drugs the woman has used, ask Question 2 for each drug/alcohol in the column and then ask Question 3 for each drug/alcohol in the column.
  - Confirm the woman's primary substance of concern.
  - If time is tight or there are many current drugs, ask Questions 4, 5, and 6 only for the primary substances of concern rather than for every drug in the column.

Table A.1. Lifetime Drug Use Chart

Over your lifetime have you ever used . . . (drug)?

Drug class	1. Ever used drug class? (Yes/No/Don't Know)	2. How many times did you use in the past year? (# of days [0–365])	3. How many times did you use in the past month? (# of days [0–31])	4. How many times have you used in your lifetime? (# of days [0–∞])	5. Start of use? (age)	6. Last use? (months, days, or years [specify])
Nicotine		# days: # times/cigs per day:	# days: # times/cigs per day:	(# years smoked)		
Alcohol						
Sedatives/hypnotics/anxiolytics (circle all that apply): Benzodiazepines, barbiturates, ludes, hits, yellow jackets, red devils						
Cannabis (note THC level if known, and # pods, cartridges, or smoking occasions per day) (hashish, hash oil)						
Stimulants (circle all that apply): Amphetamines—speed (Adderall, Ritalin), black beauties, crank, crystal, methamphetamine, speed, STP, water, yellow bam						

Drug class		1. Ever used drug class? (Yes/No/Don't Know)	2. How many times did you use in the past year? (# of days [0–365])	3. How many times did you use in the past month? (# of days [0–31])	4. How many times have you used in your lifetime? (# of days [0–∞])	5. Start of use? (age)	6. Last use? (months, days, or years [specify])
Opioids	Heroin						
	Prescription opioids (circle all that apply): OxyContin, oxycodone, Roxicodone, Tylenol with codeine, methadone, opium, morphine, Percocet, junk, fentanyl						
Cocaine							
Hallucinogens/PCP (Ecstasy, mescaline, MDA, peyote, LSD, shrooms)							
Other (circle all that apply): Inhalants (amyl & butyl nitrite, gas, glue, nitrous oxide, other solvents), steroids, antidepressants, anticonvulsants							

F. Complete SCID for DSM-5 Substance Use Disorders

The SCID-CV for DSM-5 (First et al., 2016) can be purchased from American Psychiatric Association Publishing (SET of SCID-5-CV and SCID-5-CV Users' Guide).

G. Typical Weekly Pattern Alcohol and Drug Use

Note: Use the standard drinks chart included in Session 1 of this Therapist Guide to query in enough detail to estimate the number of standard drinks per day. Write in the number of standard drinks, what time started/stopped, and also drug use, in each cell of the table. If 0, write 0.

Now I am going to ask you some more specific questions about your alcohol and drug use.

Please describe for me a usual or typical (heavy) week of drinking/drug use, over the last months leading up to your last use of alcohol or drugs. Let's start with weekdays—Monday through Friday. In a typical week, what did you normally drink or use in the morning, from the time you got up until lunchtime? (Do not include what was drunk/used with lunch. Record answers on Table A.2: Steady Pattern Chart.) *What time did you typically start and stop this use on each day?* (Write in the times.)

Now how about weekday afternoons, including what you drank or used <u>with</u> lunch, up through the afternoon until right before dinner time—what did you normally drink/use on weekday afternoons, Monday through Friday? (Record on chart.)

And how about weekday evenings? What did you normally drink/use <u>with</u> dinner, up through the rest of the evening, until the time you went to sleep? (Record on chart.)

Repeat these same instructions for weekend days, and record on the chart.

(Adapted from Miller, 1996)

Table A.2. Steady Pattern Chart: Typical Recent Week Use Pattern of Alcohol and Drugs

Week days	Morning	Afternoon	Evening	TOTAL Standard Drinks, Drugs Used, and Estimated Blood Alcohol Level
MONDAY				_____ . _____
TUESDAY				_____ . _____
WEDNESDAY				_____ . _____
THURSDAY				_____ . _____
FRIDAY				_____ . _____
SATURDAY				_____ . _____
SUNDAY				_____ . _____

H. Conduct Timeline Followback (TLFB) Interview for Daily Alcohol/Drug Use

For instructions on how to administer the TLFB (Sobell & Sobell, 1995), see Instructions for Filling Out the Timeline Alcohol Use Calendar (nova.edu) and https://www.nova.edu/gsc/forms/completing-interviewer-administered-drug-timeline-calendar.pdf. For monthly calendars, see Timeline Followback Forms and Related Materials (nova.edu).

I. Mental Health Problems/Diagnoses: Past and Current

As far as you know, have you ever been diagnosed by a mental health professional and/or physician with . . .

Problem	Yes/No	Current? Yes/No	Year Diagnosed	Treated? Basic Brief History
Depression				
Panic disorder				
Obsessive-compulsive disorder				
Trauma history or PTSD				
Generalized anxiety disorder				
Specific phobias (which one?)				
Social anxiety				
Bipolar I or II (which one?)				
Eating disorder (which one?)				
Attention-deficit/ hyperactivity disorder				
Schizophrenia, schizoaffective				
Borderline personality disorder				
Autism spectrum disorder				
Learning disability				
Other				

J. Medical Problems/Diagnoses

Do you have any current or past major medical problems or diagnoses? (Yes / No)
If yes, please describe:

_____

_____

_____

_____

K. Other Life Stressors

Are there any sources of stress that you have experienced in the last year? (Yes / No)
If yes, please describe:

_____

_____

_____

_____

L. Intimate Partner Violence Screener

Have you been hit, kicked, punched, or otherwise hurt by an intimate partner within the past year? (Yes / No)

Do you feel safe in your current relationship with your intimate partner? (Yes / No)

(From Feldhaus et al., 1997)

M. Readiness Rulers

Circle the numbers that best reflect how you are feeling about changing your alcohol/drug use or maintaining the changes you already have made:

1. How ready are you to change?

1	2	3	4	5	6	7	8	9	10

Not at all ready   Somewhat ready   Completely ready

2. How confident are you in your ability to change?

1	2	3	4	5	6	7	8	9	10

Not at all confident   Somewhat confident   Completely confident

3. How important is it to you to change?

1	2	3	4	5	6	7	8	9	10

Not at all important   Somewhat important   Completely important

References

Abulseoud, O. A., Karpyak, V. M., Schneekloth, T., Hall-Flavin, D. K., Loukianova, L. L., Geske, J. R., Biernacka, J. M., Mrazek, D. A., & Frye, M. A. (2013). A retrospective study of gender differences in depressive symptoms and risk of relapse in patients with alcohol dependence. *American Journal on Addictions*, *22*(5), 437–442.

Alvanzo, A. A., Storr, C. L., Mojtabai, R., Green, K. M., Pacek, L. R., La Flair, L. N., Cullen, B. A., & Crum, R. M. (2014). Gender and race/ethnicity differences for initiation of alcohol-related service use among persons with alcohol dependence. *Drug and Alcohol Dependence, 140*, 48–55.

American Psychiatric Association. (2013). *Diagnostic and statistical manual of mental disorders* (5th ed.). American Psychiatric Publishing.

American Psychiatric Association. (2000). *Diagnostic and statistical manual of mental disorders* (4th ed., text rev.). American Psychiatric Publishing.

Ashley, O. S., Marsden, M. E., & Brady, T. M. (2003). Effectiveness of substance abuse treatment programming for women: A review. *American Journal of Drug and Alcohol Abuse, 29*, 19–53.

Beck, A. T., & Haigh, E. (2014). Advances in cognitive theory and therapy: The generic cognitive model. *Annual Review of Clinical Psychology, 10*, 1–24.

Betty Ford Consensus Panel. (2007). What is recovery? A working definition from the Betty Ford Institute. *Journal of Substance Abuse Treatment, 33*(3), 221–228.

Bold, K. W., Epstein, E. E., & McCrady, B. S. (2017). Baseline health status and quality of life after alcohol treatment for women with alcohol dependence. *Addictive Behaviors, 64*, 35–41.

Bold, K. W., Rosen, R. L., Steinberg, M. L., Epstein, E. E., McCrady, B. S., & Williams, J. M. (2020). Smoking characteristics and alcohol use among women in treatment for alcohol use disorder. *Addictive Behaviors, 101*, 106037.

Brown, B. (2007). *I thought it was just me (but it isn't): Making the journey from "what will people think?" to "I am enough."* Avery Publishing.

Buckman, J. F., Vaschillo, B., Vaschillo, E. G., Epstein, E. E., Nguyen-Louie, T. T., Lesnewich, L. M., Eddie, D., & Bates, M. E. (2019).

Improvement in women's cardiovascular functioning during cognitive behavioral therapy for alcohol use disorder. *Psychology of Addictive Behaviors, 33*(8), 659–668.

Burns, D. (1989). *Feeling good: The new mood therapy*. William Morrow Books.

Carroll, K. (1999). Behavioral and cognitive behavioral interventions. In B. S. McCrady & E. E. Epstein (Eds.), *Addictions: A comprehensive guidebook* (pp. 250–267). Oxford University Press.

Cucciare, M. A., Simpson, T., Hoggatt, K. J., Gifford, E., & Timko, C. (2013). Substance use among women veterans: Epidemiology to evidence-based treatment. *Journal of Addictive Diseases, 32*(2), 119–139.

El-Guebaly, N. (2012). The meanings of recovery from addiction: Evolution and promises. *Journal of Addictive Medicine, 6*(1), 1–9.

Ellis, A. (1998). *How to control your anxiety before it controls you*. Kensington Publishing Corp.

Epstein, E. E., McCrady, B. S., Cook, S. N., Jensen, N., Gaba, A., Steinberg, M. L., & Bold, K. (2015). Non-ETOH drug use among women in outpatient treatment for alcohol dependence. *Drug and Alcohol Dependence, 146*, e272.

Epstein, E. E., McCrady, B. S., Hallgren, K. A., Cook, S., & Jensen, N. K., & Hildebrandt, T. (2018a). A randomized trial of female-specific cognitive behavior therapy for alcohol dependent women. *Psychology of Addictive Behaviors, 32*(1), 1–15.

Epstein, E. E., McCrady, B. S., Hallgren, K. A., Gaba, A., Cook, S., Jensen, N. K., Hildebrandt, T., Holzhauer, C., & Litt, M. (2018b). Individual versus group female-specific cognitive behavior therapy for alcohol use disorder. *Journal of Substance Abuse Treatment, 88*, 27–43.

Epstein, E. E., & Menges, D. (2013). Women and addiction. In B. S. McCrady & E. E. Epstein (Eds.), *Addictions: A comprehensive guidebook* (2nd ed., pp. 788–818). Oxford University Press.

Epstein, N. B., Werlinich, C. A., & LaTaillade, J. J. (2015). Couple therapy for partner aggression. In A. S. Gurman, J. L. Lebow, & D. K. Snyder (Eds.), *Clinical handbook of couple therapy* (5th ed., pp. 389–411). Guilford Press.

Feldhaus, K. M., Koziol-McLain, J., Amsbury, H. L., Norton, I. M., Lowenstein, S. R., & Abbott, J. T. (1997). Accuracy of 3 brief screening questions for detecting partner violence in the emergency department. *Journal of the American Medical Association, 277*(17), 1357–1361.

First, M. B., Williams, J. B. W., Karg, R. L., & Spitzer, R. L. (2016). *Structured Clinical Interview for DSM-5 Disorders, Clinician Version*. American Psychiatric Association.

Flores-Bonilla, A., & Richardson, H. N. (2020). Sex differences in the neurobiology of alcohol use disorder. *Alcohol Research: Current Review, 40*(2), 04.

Frederic, J., Sautter, F. J., Glynn, S. M., Cretu, J. B., & Senturk, D. (2015). Efficacy of structured approach therapy in reducing PTSD in returning veterans: A randomized clinical trial. *Psychological Services, 12*(3), 199–212.

Grant, B. F., Goldstein, R. B., Saha, T. D., Chou, P., Jung, J., Zhang, H., Pickering, R. P., Ruan, J., Smith, S. M., Huang, B., & Hasin, D. S. (2015). Epidemiology of DSM-5 alcohol use disorder: Results from the National Epidemiologic Survey on Alcohol and Related Conditions III. *JAMA Psychiatry, 72*(8), 757–766.

Grant, B. F., Saha, T. D., Ruan, W. J., Goldstein, R. B., Chou, S. P., Jung, J., Zhang, H., Smith, S. M., Pickering, R. P., Huang, B., & Hasin, D. S. (2016). Epidemiology of DSM-5 drug use disorder: Results from the National Epidemiologic Survey on Alcohol and Related Conditions III. *JAMA Psychiatry, 73*(1), 39–47.

Greenfield, S. F., & Pirard, S. (2009). Gender-specific treatment for women with substance use disorders. In K. T. Brady, S. E. Back, & S. F. Greenfield (Eds.), *Women and addiction: A comprehensive handbook* (pp. 289–306). Guilford Press.

Grosso, J. A., Epstein, E. E., McCrady, B. S., Gaba, A., Cook, S., Backer-Fulghum, L., & Graff, F. S. (2013). Women's motivators for seeking treatment for alcohol use disorders. *Addictive Behaviors, 38*, 2236–2245.

Grundmann, J., Lotzin, A., Sehner, S., Verthein, U., Hiller, P., Hiersemann, R., Lincoln, T. M., Hillemacher, T., Schneider, B., Driessen, M., Scherbaum, N., Dotten, A. C., & Schäfer, I. (2021). Predictors of attendance in outpatient group treatment for women with posttraumatic stress disorder and substance use disorder. *Psychotherapy Research, 31*(5), 632–643.

Hall, S. M., Havassy, B. E., & Wasserman, D. A. (1991). Effects of commitment to abstinence, positive moods, stress, and coping on relapse to cocaine use. *Journal of Consulting and Clinical Psychology, 59*(4), 526.

Hallgren, K. A., Epstein, E. E., & McCrady, B. S. (2019). Changes in hypothesized mechanisms of change before and after initiating abstinence in cognitive-behavioral therapy for women with alcohol use disorder. *Behavior Therapy, 50*(6), 1030–1041.

Hallgren, K. A., McCrady, B. S., & Epstein, E. E. (2016). Trajectories of drinking urges and the initiation of abstinence during cognitive-behavioral alcohol treatment. *Addiction, 111*(5), 854–865.

Haver, B., & Gjestad, R. (2005). Phobic anxiety and depression as predictor variables for treatment outcome: A LISREL analysis on treated female alcoholics. *Nordic Journal of Psychiatry, 59*, 25–30.

Hayaki, J., Holzhauer, C., Epstein, E. E., Lorenzo, A. C., Gaba, A., Cook, S., & McCrady, B. S. (2020). Menstrual cycle phase, alcohol consumption, alcohol cravings, and mood among women in outpatient treatment for alcohol use disorder. *Psychology of Addictive Behaviors, 34*(6), 680–689.

Heslin, K. C., Gable, A., & Dobalian, A. (2015). Special services for women in substance use disorders treatment: How does the Department of Veterans Affairs compare with other providers? *Women's Health Issues, 25*(6), 666–672.

Holzhauer, C., Cucciare, M., & Epstein, E. E. (2020a). Sex and gender effects on recovery from alcohol use disorder. *Alcohol Research Current Reviews, 40*(3). https://arcr.niaaa.nih.gov/volume/40/3/sex-and-gender-effects-recovery-alcohol-use-disorder

Holzhauer, C. G., Epstein, E. E., Hayaki, J., Marinchak, J. S., McCrady, B. S., & Cook, S. M. (2017). Moderators of sudden gains after sessions addressing emotion regulation among women in treatment for alcohol use. *Journal of Substance Abuse Treatment, 83*, 1–9.

Holzhauer, C. G., Hildebrandt, T., Epstein, E. E., McCrady, B. S., Hallgren, K. A., & Cook, S. (2020b). Mechanisms of change in female-specific and gender-neutral cognitive behavioral therapy for women with alcohol use disorder. *Journal of Clinical and Consulting Psychology, 88*(6), 541–553.

Kämmerer, A. (2019). The scientific underpinnings and impacts of shame; People who feel shame readily are at risk for depression and anxiety disorders. *Scientific American.* https://www.scientificamerican.com/article/the-scientific-underpinnings-and-impacts-of-shame/

Koob, G. F. (2013). Neuroscience of addiction. In B. S. McCrady & E. E. Epstein (Eds.), *Addictions: A comprehensive guidebook* (2nd ed., pp. 17–35). Oxford University Press.

Leonard, K. E., & Homish, G. G. (2008), Predictors of heavy drinking and drinking problems over the first 4 years of marriage. *Psychology of Addictive Behaviors, 22*(1), 25–35.

Lewis, E. T., Jamison, A. L., Ghaus, S., Durazo, E. M., Frayne, S. M., Hoggatt, K. J., Bean-Mayberry, B., Timko, C., & Cucciare, M. A. (2016). Receptivity to alcohol-related care among U.S. women Veterans with alcohol misuse. *Journal of Addictive Diseases, 35*(4), 226–237.

Longabaugh, R., Magill, M., Morgenstern, J., & Huebner, R. (2013). Mechanisms of behavior change in treatment for alcohol and other drug use disorders. In B. S. McCrady & E. E. Epstein (Eds.), *Addictions: A comprehensive guidebook* (2nd ed., pp. 572–596). Oxford University Press.

Marlatt, G. A., & Gordon, J. R. (Eds.). (1985). *Relapse prevention: Maintenance strategies in the treatment of addictive behaviors.* Guilford Press.

Mastroleo, N., & Monti, P. (2013). Cognitive-behavioral treatment for addictions. In B. S. McCrady & E. E. Epstein (Eds.), *Addictions: A comprehensive guidebook* (2nd ed., pp. 391–410). Oxford University Press.

McCrady, B. S. (2004). To have but one true friend: Implications for practice of research on alcohol use disorders and social networks. *Psychology of Addictive Behaviors, 18*, 113–121.

McCrady, B. S., & Epstein, E. E. (2021). Alcohol use disorders. In D. H. Barlow (Ed.), *Clinical handbook of psychological disorders: A step-by-step treatment manual* (6th ed., pp. 555–611). Guilford Press.

McCrady, B. S., Epstein, E. E., & Fokas, K. (2020). Treatment interventions for women with alcohol use disorder. *Alcohol Research Current Reviews, 40*(2). https://arcr.niaaa.nih.gov/volume/40/2/treatment-interventions-women-alcohol-use-disorder

McCrady, B. S., Epstein, E. E., Hallgren, K. A., Cook, S., & Jensen, N. K. (2016). Women with alcohol dependence: A randomized trial of couple versus individual plus couple therapy. *Psychology of Addictive Behaviors, 30*, 287–299.

McHugh, R. K., Votaw, V. R., Sugarman, D. E., & Greenfield, S. F. (2018). Sex and gender differences in substance use disorders. *Clinical Psychology Review, 66*, 12–23.

Miller, W. R. (1996). *Form 90: A structured assessment interview for drinking and related behaviors, test manual.* Project MATCH Monograph Series v. 5 (NIH Publication No. 96–4004). National Institute on Alcohol Abuse and Alcoholism.

Miller, W. R., & Rollnick, S. (2013). *Motivational interviewing: Helping people change* (3rd ed.). Guilford Press.

National Institute on Alcohol Abuse and Alcoholism. (2017). *Strategic plan 2017–2021.* www.nih.gov

National Institute on Alcohol Abuse and Alcoholism. (2021a). *Drinking levels defined.* https://www.niaaa.nih.gov/alcohol-health/overview-alcohol-consumption/moderate-binge-drinking

National Institute on Alcohol Abuse and Alcoholism. (2021b). *Understanding alcohol use disorder.* https://www.niaaa.nih.gov/sites/default/files/publications/Alcohol_Use_Disorder_0.pdf, p. 1.

National Institute on Drug Abuse. (2019). *The science of drug use and addiction: The basics.* https://www.drugabuse.gov/publications/media-guide/science-drug-use-addiction-basics

National Institute on Drug Abuse. (2020). *Substance use in women research report*: Summary. https://nida.nih.gov/publications/research-reports/substance-use-in-women/summary

National Survey on Drug Using Households. (2019). Section 5 PE Tables—Results from the 2019 National Survey on Drug Use and Health: Detailed Tables, SAMHSA, CBHSQ.

Neff, K., & Germer, C. (2018). *The mindful self-compassion workbook.* Guilford Press.

Olmstead, T. A., Graff, F. S., Ames-Sikora, A., McCrady, B. S., Gaba, A., & Epstein, E. E. (2019). Cost-effectiveness of individual versus group female-specific cognitive behavioral therapy for alcohol use disorder. *Journal of Substance Abuse Treatment, 100,* 1–7.

Roman, P. (2013). Treatment for substance use disorders in the United States: An organizational technology perspective. In B. S. McCrady & E. E. Epstein (Eds.), *Addictions: A comprehensive guidebook* (2nd ed., pp. 597–621). Oxford University Press.

Rosenthal, R. N. (2013). Treatment of persons with substance use disorder and co-occurring other mental disorders. In B. S. McCrady & E. E. Epstein (Eds.), *Addictions: A comprehensive guidebook* (2nd ed., pp. 659–707). Oxford University Press.

Sautter, F. J., Armelie, A. P., Glynn, S. M., & Wielt, D. B. (2011). The development of a couple-based treatment for PTSD in returning veterans. *Professional Psychology: Research and Practice, 42*(1), 63–69.

Sautter, F. J., Glynn, S. M., Cretu, J. B., Senturk, D., & Vaught, A. S. (2015). Efficacy of structured approach therapy in reducing PTSD in returning veterans: A randomized clinical trial. *Psychological Services, 12*(3), 199–212.

Sobell, L. C., & Sobell, M. B. (1995). *Alcohol Timeline Followback users' manual.* Addiction Research Foundation.

Sobell, L. C., & Sobell, M. B. (2011). *Group therapy for substance use disorders.* Guilford Press.

Substance Abuse and Mental Health Services Administration. (2009). *Substance abuse treatment: Addressing the specific needs of women.* Treatment Improvement Protocol (TIP) Series, No. 51. HHS Publication No. (SMA) 13-4426.

Timko, C., Finney, J. W., & Moos, R. H. (2005). The 8-year course of alcohol abuse: Gender differences in social context and coping. *Alcoholism: Clinical and Experimental Research, 29*(4), 612–621.

Valeri, L., Sugarman, D. E., Reilly, M. E., McHugh, R. K., Fitzmaurice, G. M., & Greenfield, S. F. (2018). Group therapy for women with substance use disorders: In-session affiliation predicts women's substance use treatment outcomes. *Journal of Substance Abuse Treatment, 94*, 60–68.

Velasquez, M. M., & Stotts, A. L. A. (2003). Substance abuse and dependence disorders in women. In M. Kopala & M. Keitel (Eds.), *Handbook of counseling women* (pp. 482–505). Sage Publications.

Volkow, N. D., & Koob, G. F. (2019). Drug addiction: The neurobiology of motivation gone awry. In S. C. Miller, D. A. Fiellin, R. N. Rosenthal, & R. Saitz (Eds.), *ASAM principles of addiction medicine* (6th ed., pp. 3–23). Lippincott Williams & Wilkins.

Walitzer, K. S., & Dearing, R. L. (2006). Gender differences in alcohol and substance use relapse. *Clinical Psychology Review, 26*(2), 128–148.

Weathers, F. W., Litz, B. T., Keane, T. M., Palmieri, P. A., Marx, B. P., & Schnurr, P. P. (2013). The PTSD Checklist for *DSM-5* (PCL-5). Scale available from the National Center for PTSD at www.ptsd.va.gov.

White, A. M. (2020). Gender difference in the epidemiology of alcohol use and related harms in the United States. *Alcohol Research: Current Reviews, 40*, 1–13.

Witkiewitz, K., & Tucker, J. A. (2020). Abstinence not required: Expanding the definition of recovery from alcohol use disorder. *Alcoholism: Clinical and Experimental Research, 44*(1), 36.

Yalom, D. (2005). *The theory and practice of group psychotherapy* (5th ed.). Basic Books.

Zweig, R. D., McCrady, B. S., & Epstein, E. E. (2009). Investigation of the psychometric properties of the Drinking Patterns Questionnaire. *Addictive Disorders & Their Treatment, 8*(1), 39–51.

Dr. Elizabeth Epstein is Professor of Psychiatry at the University of Massachusetts Chan Medical School, and Professor Emerita at the Center of Alcohol Studies (CAS), Rutgers University. Previously, Dr. Epstein was a faculty member of Rutgers CAS, most recently as Research Professor and Director of the Clinical Division of CAS with appointments at the Rutgers Graduate School of Applied and Professional Psychology and Department of Psychology. She has developed and tested numerous treatment modalities (group, couple, family, individual, telehealth) and subpopulation-specific cognitive behavioral therapy (CBT) and motivational enhancement therapy (CBT/MET) protocols for drinking and drug use problems via randomized trials funded by the National Institutes of Health. She has been or is Principal Investigator (PI), co-PI or co-investigator on NIH or VA grants to develop evidence-based CBT addiction and comorbid psychiatric treatments tailored for: women with AUD; female Veterans with AUD; couples and families; military and Veteran populations; deaf individuals; smoking cessation; opiates and chronic pain; smartphone apps for behavioral couple/family therapy; and wrap-around models of community linkage and peer support. Her addiction treatment development research program includes investigation of active ingredients, mediators, and moderators of change; as well as implementation science components to optimize dissemination and usability for broader systems of addiction care. As a licensed psychologist, Dr. Epstein has regularly provided direct clinical services to clients since 1995.

Dr. Barbara McCrady is Distinguished Professor (Emerita), University of New Mexico (UNM). Former Director of the UNM Center on Alcohol, Substance Use, and Addictions; previously at Rutgers University (1983–2007) where she served as Director of Clinical training, Chair, Department of Psychology and Clinical Director, Rutgers Center of Alcohol Studies. She was on faculty at the Brown University School of Medicine 1975–1983 where she developed and ran addictions treatment programs and conducted research. Her research focuses on empirically supported treatments for substance use disorder (SUD), including studies of: effectiveness and cost-effectiveness of cognitive-behavioral SUD treatment; conjoint treatment for persons with SUD and their spouses; Alcoholics Anonymous; alternative treatment models for women and with alcohol and other SUDs; mechanisms of change in behavioral treatments; understanding and treating SUD for persons in the criminal justice system, understanding behavioral and neurocognitive mechanisms of change in alcohol treatment. Her research has been funded by the National Institutes of Health (NIH) since 1979 and she was the PI of NIAAA pre- and post-doctoral NIH institutional research training grants at Rutgers and UNM (1994–2021). She has served as President of Division 50 (Addictions) of the American Psychological Association, President of the Research Society on Alcoholism, and Secretary-Treasurer of the Association for Behavioral and Cognitive Therapies.